CW01631258

HIP PAIN RELIEF & STRENGTH

Exercises to Restore Mobility, Reduce Chronic Hip Pain, and Protect Your Back and Knees

By Evan Calder

This book is a work of nonfiction. While the stories shared are inspired by real experiences, some names and identifying details have been changed to protect privacy.

This book is intended for educational and informational purposes and reflects general movement, fitness, and rehabilitation principles. It is not intended to diagnose, treat, cure, or prevent any medical condition, nor is it a substitute for professional medical advice, physical therapy, or other qualified healthcare services.

Your health and safety matter. If at any point you feel unsure, experience increasing pain, or have concerns about your condition, pause and seek guidance from a qualified professional who can provide care tailored to your needs.

Published by Edenroot Press
edenrootpress.com

EDENROOT
PRESS

Contents

About Evan Calder

Evan Calder is a movement and recovery educator specializing in injury rehabilitation, physical resilience, and long-term strength for everyday people. His work focuses on helping readers rebuild confidence in their bodies after pain, injury, illness, or major life changes, without relying on extremes, shortcuts, or fear-based advice.

Over the past decade, Evan has worked at the intersection of fitness training, rehabilitation principles, and behavior change, helping thousands of people recover from chronic pain, return to activity after injury, and regain independence through structured, progressive movement. His approach blends modern exercise science, physical therapy concepts, and practical coaching into clear, step-by-step systems that readers can safely follow at home.

What sets Evan's work apart is his emphasis on **understanding before effort**. Rather than prescribing endless exercises, he teaches readers *why* pain persists, *how* the body adapts, and *when* to progress or pull back. His programs are designed to reduce fear, rebuild trust in movement, and create sustainable results, especially for people who feel stuck, frustrated, or overwhelmed by conflicting advice.

Evan's writing is informed by years of hands-on experience with individuals recovering from back pain, joint injuries, nerve pain, post-surgical limitations, stroke, postpartum changes, and training-related setbacks. He is especially known for translating complex rehabilitation ideas into simple routines, clear progressions, and realistic plans that fit real lives.

The **Recovery Series** reflects Evan's core belief: Healing happens when calm, consistency, and intelligent progression replace urgency and guesswork. Each book in the series follows a structured framework that helps readers calm pain, restore mobility, rebuild strength, and return confidently to daily life or sport, with prevention strategies built in from the start.

Evan lives quietly, trains consistently, and continues to study how people heal best when they are given clarity, patience, and a system they can trust.

Acknowledgements

This book is for the people who keep moving even when movement has become complicated.

To the readers who've lived through the quiet frustration of hip pain, having to think about stairs, long walks, getting out of a car, or rolling over in bed, thank you for trusting a process that values patience over panic. Your willingness to rebuild slowly is not "less athletic." It's the most durable kind of strength.

To the desk workers who learned that sitting isn't a moral failure but a position that needs balancing, thank you for choosing small movement interrupts instead of all-or-nothing resets. Those small reps change bodies.

To the walkers, hikers, and everyday movers who discovered that "just walking" is training when it's dosed properly, thank you for practicing baseline, restraint, and consistency. The hip responds to the steady rhythm more than it responds to intensity.

To the runners and lifters who returned to training without trying to prove anything, thank you for letting the plan lead. Choosing a run/walk baseline, lowering a box squat, reducing load for cleaner reps, those choices are how careers and bodies last.

To the clinicians, researchers, and educators who continue to refine how we understand pain, load, adaptation, and recovery, thank you for building the foundation that makes practical guidance possible. Translating science into daily decisions is a shared craft, and this book stands on that collective work.

To the patients and clients I've learned from across years of coaching and rehab education: the ones who taught me that fear is rarely solved by more information alone, and that confidence is built through repeated safe experiences, thank you. The best systems are shaped by real people, not theories.

To the people behind the scenes who make steady work possible, editors, designers, proofreaders, and anyone who helps turn a clear idea into a finished book, thank you for your precision and patience. Clarity is a team effort.

And finally: thank you to anyone who has ever felt behind, broken, or uncertain and still chose to take the next calm step. If this book helped you replace urgency with a plan, if it helped you trade guesswork for a baseline and progressions, then it has done its job.

Evan Calder

Chapter 1: Why Hip Pain Affects the Whole Body

What will improve when you understand the "chain"

You'll stop treating the hip like an isolated joint and start managing **load** across the system.

You'll recognize compensation patterns (back stiffness, knee ache, limping) as **strategies**, not failures.

You'll learn why **single-leg control** is the quiet foundation beneath walking, stairs, running, and lifting.

You'll know what to change first: not everything, just the few levers that reduce irritation and build capacity.

The hip's real job (and why it's a big deal)

Your hip is not just a hinge. It's a deep ball-and-socket joint designed to:

Accept load from the ground (walking, stairs, running)

Transfer load to the pelvis and spine

Create stability when you're on one leg (most of life)

Generate power when needed (standing up, sprinting, lifting)

When hip tissues get irritated, tendons, joint surfaces, bursa, surrounding muscle, your system often shifts load to other areas that can "help" in the short term. The body is clever. It will borrow motion from your low back, or borrow stability from your knee, or borrow rotation from your foot. That borrowing keeps you moving, but it can raise irritation elsewhere.

The goal of this book is not to shame those strategies. The goal is to **give your body better options**.

The chain reaction map: hip → pelvis → back → knee

Here are three common pathways. You may recognize one, or a blend.

Pathway 1: Hip stiffness → low back "helping"

If the hip doesn't rotate or extend well (often noticed when walking uphill, standing from a chair, or running), the pelvis may tilt or rotate differently. The low back might move more to compensate, especially during long sitting-to-standing days. That can create a pattern where the back feels tight or "jammed," even though the hip is the quieter driver.

Translation: Sometimes "back pain" is the back doing extra work because the hip isn't sharing the job.

Pathway 2: Hip weakness → knee managing alignment

When the hip muscles fatigue, especially the glutes and deep rotators, your knee may drift inward during stairs, lunges, or running (a common single-leg control issue). The knee is a hardworking joint, but it doesn't love being the primary controller of pelvis position. Over time, knee tissues can get irritated.

Translation: The knee often complains when it's asked to stabilize what the hip should stabilize.

Pathway 3: Hip irritation → stride changes → more load per step

If a step hurts, you instinctively shorten stride, shift weight early, rotate the foot out, or lean the trunk. Those are sensible "get through the day" tactics. But they change how force travels through the chain. You may end up with:

- More impact on the other hip
- More tension in the front of the hip (hip flexor/adductor overload)
- More stiffness in the low back
- More knee compression from altered alignment

Translation: Pain changes mechanics; mechanics change load; load influences pain.

This isn't a doom loop. It's a map. Maps are useful because they show you where to intervene.

The lever we'll train first: repeatable single-leg control

Most of life is single-leg: walking, stairs, changing direction, stepping off a curb. Even standing "on two legs" is often one leg doing more. When single-leg control improves, the hip stops feeling like a fragile hinge and starts feeling like a reliable foundation.

Single-leg control is not about squeezing every muscle. It's about **stacking** and **sharing** load:

Foot contacts the ground without gripping

Knee tracks in a steady line (not rigid, not collapsing)

Hip stays level enough without hiking or dumping

Trunk stays calm without dramatic side bending

We will build this through phases: foundational stability → single-leg control → load and power. But we start with a basic rule: **control comes before intensity.**

Your symptom-guided training rules (simple, not fragile)

You're going to see this logic throughout the book. Start using it now.

Rule 1: Train inside tolerance, not inside fear

Acceptable: mild discomfort (0–3/10) that feels non-sharp and improves as you warm up

Not acceptable: sharp pain, catching, giving way, or pain that forces you to limp
If you change your gait, you've exceeded today's dose.

Rule 2: 24-hour check

After a session, you should return close to baseline within 24 hours. If you're noticeably worse the next day (more limp, less range, more night sensitivity), regress the next session by reducing:

Range of motion

Load (weight/band tension)

Volume (sets/reps)

Speed (slow it down)
Pick **one** variable first. Don't delete movement entirely unless symptoms demand it.

Rule 3: Build capacity with small, frequent wins

Hip pain often improves faster with "low-to-moderate doses" repeated consistently than with occasional hard workouts. Think **minimum effective dose**, not maximum effort.

A good starting template (we'll refine later):

Mobility: 5–10 minutes most days

Strength: 2–4 days/week

Walking: a tolerable daily baseline (even short)

Rule 4: Irritation vs injury language

This matters because it changes behavior.

Irritation: sensitive tissues, often dose-related, improves with smarter loading and time

Injury: significant structural damage or acute trauma, often requires evaluation and different pacing
Many people have irritation with protective movement, not a catastrophic injury. Your job is to respond with calm structure.

Real-life examples (so you can stop guessing)

Desk worker with stiff, achy hip

Pattern: feels worse after sitting, first steps are stiff, improves after moving.

First move: short mobility "interrupts" + foundational strength.
Decision rule: If sitting is the trigger, don't stretch harder at night, add small movement earlier in the day to reduce irritation buildup.

Walker who gets sore on longer walks

Pattern: fine at 10 minutes, sore at 30, flares at 45.
First move: set a **walking baseline** at 10–15 minutes, then add strength to raise capacity.
Decision rule: Increase walk time by 10–20% only when next-day symptoms stay near baseline.

Runner with lateral hip pain

Pattern: pain during or after runs, especially hills/speed, sometimes knee ache.
First move: reduce run load temporarily, train single-leg control and hip endurance, then reintroduce running with rules.
Decision rule: If pain increases during the run and changes stride, stop and swap to walking + later-phase return plan.

Lifter who feels pinching in deep squats

Pattern: deep hip flexion sensitivity, sometimes groin ache.
First move: adjust range, train hip control through tolerable depth, strengthen glutes/adductors in safer positions.

Decision rule: Range is a variable. Keep training, just choose a depth that respects tolerance.

The traps that keep hip pain "stuck" (and the better option)

Trap 1: Chasing a perfect diagnosis before taking safe action

Better: Use red flags to rule out urgency, then begin conservative, symptom-guided loading. Clarity often increases *after* the system calms down.

Trap 2: Stretching harder when the hip is irritated

Better: If stretching causes lingering soreness, shift to **gentle mobility** + **isometrics** + controlled strength. Mobility is an input; your response is the data.

Trap 3: Training only the painful spot

Better: Train the chain. Foot/ankle tolerance, knee alignment, trunk control, and walking mechanics all affect hip load.

Trap 4: Rest-only after every flare-up

Better: Use step-down rules (later chapters) to keep movement present, just scaled. Capacity hates long gaps.

Today's Action Plan (simple and specific)

Use this checklist immediately.

Set your baseline: What can you do today that doesn't spike symptoms tomorrow? (Walk time, stairs, sit-to-stand.)

Pick one daily mobility slot: 5 minutes, same time each day. Consistency beats intensity.

Choose one strength anchor: 2–3 exercises you can do without sharp pain (we'll build your menu in upcoming chapters).

Use the 24-hour check: If next day is worse, regress one variable (range, load, volume, speed).

Watch your limp: If you limp, your dose is too high today. Scale it.

Your hip doesn't need you to be brave. It needs you to be consistent.

Chapter 2: Acute vs Chronic Hip Pain

What this chapter will change for you

- You'll learn to sort your symptoms into **acute** vs **persistent** patterns without panic.
- You'll understand "**irritation vs injury**" in practical terms and what it means for training.
- You'll get clear **decision rules** for what to do in the first 72 hours vs the next 3–6 weeks.
- You'll stop treating every flare as damage, and start treating it as **dose feedback**.

Two timelines, two strategies

Hip pain often gets confusing because we mix timelines. Acute pain and chronic pain can feel similar in the moment (especially if you're worried), but they respond best to different approaches.

Acute (new or recently aggravated) hip pain

Usually: **0–6 weeks**, often with a clear trigger, new training load, long walk, awkward lift, deep squat day, sudden sprint, long drive, a slip, a fall, or "I woke up and it's angry."

Acute pain is often dominated by **irritability**: the tissues and nervous system are sensitive and reactive. Your job is not to "fix everything." Your job is to **calm the system and reintroduce load safely**.

Chronic (persistent or recurring) hip pain

Usually: **6+ weeks**, or pain that keeps returning for months/years. Sometimes it started as acute pain and never fully settled; other times it crept in gradually.

Persistent pain is often dominated by **capacity mismatch**: your hip is being asked to do more than it's currently conditioned for, especially in single-leg tasks, stairs, hills, running, deep flexion, or long sitting days.

Your job here is to **rebuild capacity**: strength, tolerance, movement options, and confidence.

Irritation vs injury: a calmer way to think

These are not medical diagnoses. They're working categories that guide behavior.

"Irritation" patterns (common, often load-related)

- Symptoms vary day to day
- Often improves with warming up or gentle movement
- More sensitive after spikes in activity (long walk, hills, deep squats, long sitting)
- Feels achy, tight, or “worked,” sometimes sharp briefly but not consistently
- Responds to **dose adjustment** and gradual strengthening

Common examples: tendinopathy-type irritation, bursa irritation, muscular overload, joint sensitivity, movement protection.

“Injury” patterns (more concerning, needs clarity)

- Clear trauma (fall, collision, forced twist)
- Sudden inability to bear weight, giving way, or severe swelling/bruising
- Pain that is sharp and constant with major loss of function
- Symptoms that rapidly worsen without clear cause

Mechanical symptoms that are new and significant (locking, true catching with collapse)

Red flags (fever, unexplained weight loss, night pain that escalates, neurological changes)

This book helps with conservative rehab. If you suspect injury, get assessed.

The first question: “How reactive is it?” (irritability scale)

Instead of obsessing over labels, use an irritability check. Rate your hip today:

Low irritability

Pain is mild and predictable

You can walk normally

Symptoms settle quickly after activity

You can tolerate controlled strength work

Moderate irritability

Pain is noticeable and limits some tasks (stairs, hills, deep bending)

Symptoms linger for hours after activity

You may have mild gait changes if you push it

Strength is possible but needs careful dosing and shorter ranges

High irritability

Pain is easily triggered

You limp or avoid weight-bearing

Night pain is prominent or sleep is disrupted

Many movements feel “hot” or threatening

Even small increases in activity spike symptoms

Your strategy is matched to irritability, not your willpower.
High irritability = calm it down first. Low irritability = build.

Acute flare or fresh pain: what to do in the first 72 hours

The goal is to reduce threat, keep circulation, and prevent the "freeze."

Step 1: Protect without parking

Avoid what clearly spikes symptoms (deep hip flexion, long hills, heavy lunges, long sitting). But keep **gentle movement** present.

A simple 10-minute "keep it moving" set (1–2x/day):

- Easy walk: 3–7 minutes (flat)
- Hip-friendly range: 1–2 drills from Chapter 5/6 later (gentle)
- Light isometrics (no sharp pain): 2–3 sets of 20–30 seconds

If walking hurts immediately or you can't bear weight, that's not a "push through" moment, seek evaluation.

Step 2: Use pain as a boundary, not a bully

During movement: keep discomfort **0–3/10** and non-sharp.
After movement: symptoms should settle toward baseline within **24 hours**.

If you're worse tomorrow, scale back one variable:

- Less range
- Less time
- Fewer sets
- Slower tempo

Step 3: Don't gamble with aggressive stretching

In acute irritability, long aggressive stretches can increase protective tone. Prefer **short, gentle mobility** and **controlled activation**.

Persistent hip pain: the 3-part model that usually works

Chronic pain tends to respond to a layered approach:

Layer 1: Restore options (mobility that "earns" range)

Not maximum flexibility, useful range that you can control. The assessment in Chapter 6 will show what matters for you.

Layer 2: Build local capacity (hip muscles that share load)

Glute strength, adductor support, and hip flexor tolerance, without compensation patterns. Chapters 7–9 guide this.

Layer 3: Rebuild global function (walking, stairs, running, lifting)

Your hip must perform inside real tasks. Chapters 10–15 and the phase training do this.

This model works because it respects the whole chain: hip function reduces the need for back/knee compensation.

A practical sorting tool: which "bucket" are you in?

Use this quick screen. Choose the closest fit:

Bucket A: Fresh and sensitive (acute/high irritability)

New pain or sudden flare

Walking is limited or limping appears

Night discomfort is higher than usual

Best next step: Chapter 3 for safety, then Chapter 5 (7-day relief) before heavy strength.

Bucket B: Annoying but manageable (acute/moderate irritability)

Triggered by a known load change

You can walk mostly normally

Symptoms settle with pacing

Best next step: Start Chapter 5 plan, then begin Phase 1 strength in Chapter 11.

Bucket C: Persistent pattern (chronic/low-to-moderate irritability)

Recurring or lasting 6+ weeks

Worse with certain tasks (stairs, sitting, running)

No major trauma, no red flags

Best next step: Chapter 6 assessment + Phase training (11–13) alongside walking mechanics.

Bucket D: Unclear or concerning

Rapid worsening, systemic signs, new neurological symptoms, inability to bear weight, major trauma
Best next step: Chapter 3 and seek evaluation.

Buckets can change week to week. That's normal.

The mistakes that prolong hip pain (and the steadier alternative)

Mistake 1: Treating acute pain like a fitness test

Instead: In the first week, focus on *calm exposure*, small doses, frequent wins.

Mistake 2: Treating chronic pain like a rest problem

Instead: Most persistent hip pain improves with **progressive loading**. Rest can calm a flare, but it won't build capacity.

Mistake 3: Changing everything at once

Instead: Change one lever, observe 24 hours, then adjust. This keeps your plan measurable.

Mistake 4: Overvaluing "tightness" as the main cause

Instead: Tight can be protective tone from irritation or weakness. Often the winning combo is **mobility + strength**, not stretching alone.

Mistake 5: Waiting for zero pain before training

Instead: Train inside tolerance. Pain-free isn't required; *stable and improving* is the goal.

Decision rules: progress, hold, regress

Use these rules starting today.

Progress (add a small challenge) when:

- Symptoms are stable or improving for **3–5 days**
- No increase in limp
- Next-day soreness returns near baseline
- You feel more confident in daily tasks

Progress options (pick one):

- Add 1 set
- Add 2–5 reps per set

Add a small load

Increase range slightly

Add a slightly harder variation

Hold (keep the same dose) when:

Symptoms fluctuate but stay within baseline range

You're adapting to a new exercise

Sleep or stress is high (recovery capacity down)

Regress (scale down) when:

Pain increases to **5+/10** during training

You limp during/after

Next day is clearly worse

Night pain increases beyond your normal pattern

Regress options (pick one):

Reduce range first

- Reduce volume second
- Reduce load third
- Slow tempo or add pauses
- Swap to isometrics for 3–7 days

Quick checklist: your next best step

- Identify your timeline: **fresh flare** or **persistent pattern**
- Rate irritability: low / moderate / high
- Choose the matching strategy: calm exposure vs capacity building
- Use the 24-hour check to steer dose
- If symptoms are severe, traumatic, rapidly worsening, or unclear: move to **Chapter 3**

Chapter 3: When Hip Pain Needs Medical Care

What this chapter will change for you

- You'll know the **specific signs** that should override "wait and see."
- You'll learn the difference between "**worth checking**" and "**urgent**."
- You'll get a simple **triage script** for booking the right type of care.
- You'll understand which symptoms mean "pause training" vs "scale training."

The goal: calm clarity, not catastrophizing

Most hip pain is not dangerous. But some patterns deserve prompt evaluation, because missing them can delay appropriate care, and because pushing through the wrong situation can worsen outcomes.

This chapter is your filter. Think of it as a safety net: you may never need it, but having it reduces fear and guesswork.

The "stop sign" symptoms (urgent evaluation)

Seek urgent medical care (urgent care / emergency services depending on severity) if you have any of the following:

1) You can't bear weight or you suddenly collapse

You cannot take **four steps** without severe pain or giving way

You feel the leg won't support you, or you're unable to stand from a chair

Why it matters: This can signal fracture, significant structural injury, severe joint inflammation, or neurological compromise. Don't "test it again tomorrow."

2) Significant trauma or a fall, especially with osteoporosis risk

Fall from height, car accident, collision sports impact

Or a lower-level fall if you're older, have osteoporosis, or use long-term steroids

Why it matters: Hip and pelvic fractures can be subtle early but worsen with continued loading.

3) Fever, chills, redness/warmth, or you feel systemically unwell

- Hip pain plus fever or a hot swollen joint
- Recent infection, injection, surgery, or immune suppression increases concern

Why it matters: Joint infection is uncommon but serious and needs prompt assessment.

4) Rapid swelling, severe bruising, or a hot swollen limb

- Sudden large swelling around hip/thigh
- Calf swelling with pain, warmth, or shortness of breath/chest pain

Why it matters: This raises concern for bleeding/hematoma, severe tissue injury, or clot-related issues.

5) New neurological red flags

Progressive numbness, weakness, or loss of coordination

New bowel/bladder changes

Severe back pain with spreading neurological symptoms

Why it matters: This can signal significant nerve or spinal involvement requiring urgent care.

6) Severe night pain that is escalating and not position-related

Pain that wakes you repeatedly and keeps escalating

Especially if it's accompanied by systemic signs (fever, weight loss)

Why it matters: While night pain can happen with benign issues, escalating non-mechanical night pain deserves timely evaluation.

The "yellow flag" patterns (book an appointment soon)

These situations are not necessarily emergencies, but they do deserve professional assessment, especially if they're new or persistent.

1) Pain that is steadily worsening over 1–2 weeks despite conservative care

If your activity is stable (you're not suddenly doing more) and pain is still climbing, get checked.

2) Persistent inability to return to baseline walking

If you've had **more than 7–10 days** of altered gait or limping, it's worth an assessment. Limping is a big load modifier.

3) True mechanical symptoms that change function

- Locking (you literally can't move the hip briefly)
- Catching that causes the leg to "give way"
- Sharp, consistent groin pain with specific ranges that doesn't soften with regressions

These can be joint-related and deserve clarity. Many clicks/pops are harmless; what matters is **loss of function** and **reliably provoking sharp pain**.

4) Significant pain in high-risk groups

Extra caution if you are:

- Older (especially 60+)
- Osteoporotic or at risk (history, family history, steroid use)
- Have known inflammatory arthritis
- Have a history of cancer
- Recently postpartum with new severe hip/groin pain (rare issues exist; don't ignore severe symptoms)

5) Pain with unexplained weight loss, fatigue, or persistent malaise

Not common, but it's a "check sooner" pattern.

"But what if it's arthritis / labrum / bursitis?"

Labels can be helpful, but they can also create fear.

A few grounding points:

- Imaging findings (like "degeneration" or "labral changes") are common, even in people without pain.

Many hip pain patterns improve with **conservative loading**, even when imaging shows changes.

Your plan doesn't depend on a perfect label; it depends on:

- red flags ruled out
- irritability managed
- capacity rebuilt

If a clinician gives you a diagnosis, use it as information, not a life sentence.

When to pause training vs scale training

A lot of people swing between two extremes: "do nothing" or "push through." Here's the middle path.

Pause training (and seek care) if:

- You can't bear weight
- There is recent trauma + severe pain

Pain is rapidly worsening

You have fever/systemic signs

New neurological symptoms appear

The hip feels unstable in a new, alarming way

Scale training (keep movement, reduce dose) if:

Symptoms are clearly load-related

Pain is moderate but predictable

You can walk without a significant limp

Symptoms settle toward baseline within 24 hours

No red flags are present

Scaling means: less range, less load, fewer sets, slower tempo, and more isometrics.

The "4-step triage" you can use today

If you're unsure what to do, run this sequence:

Step 1: Can you bear weight normally?

Yes: proceed to Step 2

No / limping severely: seek evaluation now

Step 2: Any systemic signs? (fever, chills, feeling ill)

Yes: seek evaluation now

No: proceed to Step 3

Step 3: Any major trauma or high-risk factors?

Yes: book urgent assessment

No: proceed to Step 4

Step 4: Is it improving with conservative dosing over 7–10 days?

Yes: continue plan with symptom-guided progression

No / worsening: book an appointment

This keeps you grounded in reality, not anxiety.

How to talk to a clinician (so you're taken seriously and you get answers)

When you book an appointment, you can describe your symptoms in a way that leads to better decisions. Use this simple structure:

Timeline: "This started on ___ and has been present for ___ days/weeks."

Trigger: "It began after ___ (run, long drive, new lifting program, fall)."

Location: "The main pain is ___ (groin/front, side, buttock, radiating)."

Function: "I can/can't bear weight; stairs are ___; walking is limited to ___ minutes."

Irritability: "It worsens with ___ and settles in ___ hours."

Red flags: "No fever/weight loss/neurological symptoms" (or state if present).

Goal: "I want a conservative plan and guidance on safe loading."

If you want imaging, ask a better question than "Do I need an MRI?" Try:

“What diagnoses are you considering, and would imaging change the plan?”
That keeps care aligned with decisions, not just curiosity.

The most common fear: “Am I making it worse?”

In most non-red-flag cases, **gentle, symptom-guided movement does not worsen tissue health**. It often improves it. The risk isn’t movement, it’s **overdose** (too much range/load/volume too soon) or **ignoring stop signs**.

Your safest path is:

- check for red flags
- set a baseline
- rebuild capacity gradually
- use the 24-hour check as your guardrail

That’s what the next chapters give you.

Action plan: your safety checklist

✅ No red flags (weight-bearing, systemic signs, neuro changes)

✅ Pain is dose-related and settles within 24 hours

✅ You can walk without a meaningful limp

✅ You can begin conservative mobility + isometrics (Ch.5)

✅ If not improving by 7–10 days, or worsening: book an assessment

Chapter 4: The Sitting and Overuse Problem

What this chapter will change for you

You'll understand why hip pain often isn't about one "bad movement," but about **repeated positions + repeated load**.

You'll learn how sitting changes hip behavior (stiffness, flexor/adductor sensitivity, glute "sleepiness").

You'll get a simple plan to reduce irritation without obsessing over posture: **movement interrupts + smarter dose**.

You'll know how to spot overuse patterns early and adjust before a flare-up.

The real issue: your hip adapts to what you repeat

The hip is highly adaptable. That's good news, because it means change is possible. It's also the trap: if your day repeats the same position for hours, or the same training stress for weeks, your hip will adapt to that too.

Two common drivers of hip pain in otherwise healthy people are:

- **Prolonged sitting** (long hip flexion, low movement variety)
- **Overuse** (repeated load without adequate recovery or progression)

These drivers don't make you fragile. They just narrow your hip's options until "normal life" starts feeling like too much.

Why sitting irritates hips (without needing perfect posture)

Sitting puts the hip in flexion, often 70–100 degrees, sometimes more if you sink into a soft chair. Over time, three things tend to happen:

1) You lose "easy" hip extension

Hip extension is the motion behind you, needed for walking stride, climbing stairs, and running. When you sit a lot, extension isn't practiced. The body often responds by:

- stiffening the front of the hip

borrowing extension from the low back

shortening stride without you noticing

This is one reason hip pain often comes with back tightness.

2) Hip flexors and adductors get overworked, not just "tight"

If you're in flexion all day, the tissues at the front and inner hip can become sensitive, especially if you then ask them to do a lot suddenly (hills, stairs, sprints, deep lunges).

Important nuance: what feels like "tightness" is often **protective tone** from irritation. Stretching harder can sometimes amplify it.

3) Glutes contribute less automatically

Glutes don't turn off, but their timing can change. After prolonged sitting, many people load the hip by:

shifting into the front of the hip

rotating the feet outward

using the low back more to stand up

That's not laziness. It's a predictable adaptation to repeated sitting.

Overuse: the quiet math of load vs capacity

Overuse happens when **load increases faster than capacity**. Load is not just weight in the gym. Load is:

- walking volume
- hills and stairs
- running speed, stride length, terrain
- standing time
- sleep quality (recovery)
- stress (sensitization)
- sudden changes in footwear
- new mobility work that's too aggressive

Overuse pain often shows up as:

- a predictable ache during or after activity

- tenderness on the side of the hip or deep groin discomfort
- stiffness that's worse after rest, then eases with movement
- a pattern of "fine for a few days, then flare"

The mistake is assuming that because one session caused pain, that session was "wrong." Often it was just **too much, too soon** given your current baseline.

The two common patterns (so you can identify yours)

Pattern A: The desk-day hip

- Stiff first steps after sitting
- Pain when standing from low chairs
- Relief after moving, then flare after long sitting again
  Main lever: frequent movement interrupts + gentle extension practice + glute re-engagement.

Pattern B: The active overuse hip

- Fine at the start of walks/runs, worse later or afterward
- Sensitive to hills, speed, deep ranges
- “Hot” lateral hip after longer sessions
  Main lever: set a repeatable baseline, rebuild strength capacity, reintroduce volume gradually.

Many people have both: desk-day stiffness plus weekend overuse.

Your practical system: interrupts, anchors, and dosage

You don’t need a standing desk, perfect posture, or a new life. You need three simple systems.

System 1: Movement interrupts (the anti-stiffness dose)

Every 30–60 minutes of sitting, do **1–2 minutes** of movement. That’s it.

Pick one:

- Walk to the kitchen and back

10 sit-to-stands (hands allowed)

30–60 seconds of gentle hip extension rocks (standing, small range)

5 slow "marches" per side (controlled, not high)

5–8 step-ups on a low step

Rule: Interrupts should feel easy. If an interrupt feels like a workout, it won't stick.

System 2: Daily "hip anchors" (short, consistent, repeatable)

Choose two anchors: one mobility, one strength. Total time: 8–15 minutes.

Mobility anchor (choose 1–2):

Gentle hip flexion/rotation rocks (pain-free range)

Supported hip extension drill (small range)

Adductor rock-backs (easy, not deep)

Strength anchor (choose 1–2):

- Isometric wall sit (short range) or supported split-stance hold
- Glute bridge iso holds (if tolerated)
- Side-lying abduction holds (careful to avoid hip hiking)

We'll build a full menu in Chapters 5–9. For now, the point is structure: do the same few moves often enough that your hip trusts the routine.

System 3: Dosage rules for overuse (so you stop rolling the dice)

Use these three guardrails:

Baseline first
If you flare after 30 minutes of walking, your baseline is not 30. Start at 10–15 (or whatever is repeatable).

Add slowly
When symptoms are stable for 3–5 days, increase walk/run volume by **10–20%** at most. If you're very sensitive, use 5–10%.

One change at a time
Don't increase distance and add hills and start a new strength plan in the same week. Capacity

builds fastest when the signal is clear.

Sitting doesn't require fear, just strategy

A common anxiety loop is "Sitting is ruining my hips." That story increases threat. The more useful frame is: sitting is a **position with a cost** if it's uninterrupted and unbalanced by movement variety.

You can sit. You just don't want to sit *for hours without interruption* and then demand high output from a deconditioned hip.

A realistic day might be:

Morning: 5-minute mobility anchor

Workday: 6–10 movement interrupts total

Evening: 8–12 minutes strength anchor

Walk: your baseline dose (even if short)

That's not extreme. That's intelligent repetition.

Common missteps (and steadier alternatives)

Misstep 1: "I'll fix sitting with one long stretch at night."

Instead: Use interrupts during the day. Night stretching can be optional and gentle, but it's not the main lever.

Misstep 2: Forcing deep hip stretches when the front of the hip is irritated

Instead: Reduce depth, use short-range mobility, and add isometrics. You're earning tolerance, not winning a flexibility contest.

Misstep 3: "I'll stop walking/running completely until it's perfect."

Instead: Set a baseline dose you can repeat. Movement is a key input for hip health, just dose it correctly.

Misstep 4: Training through fatigue patterns

If your hip control collapses (knee diving in, trunk leaning, foot gripping), you're no longer building capacity, you're practicing compensation.
Instead: Stop the set earlier and keep quality within tolerance.

Quick checklist / Action plan

Pick a **movement interrupt** you'll do every 30–60 minutes of sitting (1–2 minutes).

Set a walking baseline you can repeat without next-day worsening.

Choose two daily anchors: **one mobility, one strength** (8–15 minutes total).

Follow the overuse rules: baseline → slow increases → one change at a time.

If a drill increases symptoms for more than 24 hours, regress range or volume.

Your hip doesn't need dramatic solutions. It needs a steadier rhythm.

Chapter 5: 7-Day Hip Pain Relief Plan

What this chapter will change for you

- You'll have a **conservative 7-day plan** that calms symptoms without freezing your body.
- You'll learn a repeatable daily structure: **reset → restore → reinforce**.
- You'll know exactly how to scale the plan for **high vs moderate vs low irritability**.
- You'll gain confidence through clear **progress / hold / step-down rules**.

The purpose of the first week: calm the system and rebuild trust

When hip pain is loud, most people do one of two things: push through or shut down. Both tend to prolong the problem.

This 7-day plan sits in the middle: enough movement to keep the hip supplied and coordinated, but conservative enough to reduce irritation. It's designed for:

- new flare-ups
- persistent pain that's currently reactive
- anyone who feels unsure what is "safe"

Your main goal this week is **symptom stability**. Strength gains can come later. Stability first.

The structure: Reset → Restore → Reinforce

Each day has three parts. Total time: **15–25 minutes**, split if needed.

Reset (2–4 minutes)
Downshift the system and reduce protective tone.

Restore (6–10 minutes)
Gentle mobility to reintroduce motion options, without forcing end range.

Reinforce (6–12 minutes)
Low-threat strength inputs (mostly isometrics +

controlled reps) that tell the hip, "you can handle load."

Add a short walk if tolerated. Walking is a key input, just dose it.

Before you start: choose your irritability track

Use this to pick the right version.

Track A - High irritability

limping appears easily

pain feels sharp/hot or unpredictable

night pain is higher than normal

Plan: smaller ranges, more isometrics, shorter walks.

Track B - Moderate irritability

pain predictable with certain tasks

walking mostly normal if paced

Plan: full menu with conservative reps, optional

small progressions.

Track C - Low irritability

discomfort mild and stable

you mainly feel stiffness or “weakness”
Plan: add a little more controlled strength, still keep it calm.

If you’re unsure, start with Track B and adjust using the 24-hour check.

Your rules for the week (non-negotiable guardrails)

During: keep discomfort in the **0–3/10** range and non-sharp.

After: symptoms should settle toward baseline within **24 hours**.

No limping practice: if you limp, scale the dose (less range/time).

One variable at a time: if you change anything, change one thing.

The 7-Day Plan (day-by-day)

Day 1: Calm exposure (find your safe menu)

Reset (2 min)

4 slow breaths: inhale through nose, long exhale (6 8 seconds).

Gentle weight shifts side-to-side (30–60 seconds), small range.

Restore (6–8 min) *(choose 2)*

Supported hip rock-backs (hands on chair or counter)

Hinge back slightly, then return tall.

8–10 reps, slow.

90/90 support rotations (modified)

Sit on floor or firm surface, hands behind you, rotate gently side to side within comfort.

6–8 each side.

Adductor rock-backs (easy range)

On hands/knees, one leg out to side, rock back gently.

6–10 reps each side.

Reinforce (6–10 min) *(choose 2)*

Glute bridge iso (or shorter-range bridge)

3 x 20–30 sec, rest 30–45 sec.

Cue: “ribs down, push through heels, stop before hamstrings cramp.”

Wall-supported split-stance hold

One foot forward, one back, light support from wall/counter.

3 x 20 sec each side.

Cue: "front heel heavy, pelvis level, breathe."

Side-lying abduction hold *(small lift)*

2–3 x 15–25 sec each side.

Cue: "toe slightly down, don't hike the hip."

Optional walk: 5–10 minutes flat, easy.

Today's win: identify which moves reduce stiffness and which provoke symptoms.

Day 2: Repeat and smooth (same menu, cleaner execution)

Keep the same menu as Day 1 unless yesterday clearly worsened you. If worse: reduce range by 20–30% and shorten holds by 5–10 seconds.

Add one technique focus:

Move slower, and keep breath steady during isometrics.
Breath control reduces guarding.

Optional walk: same as Day 1, not more.

Day 3: Add gentle capacity (only if stable)

If you wake up near baseline, you can progress one small variable:

Choose **one**:

- add 1 set to one reinforce drill, OR
- add 2 reps to one restore drill, OR
- add 2–5 minutes to your walk

If you're not stable, keep Day 2 exactly.

Reinforce upgrade option (Track B/C):

- Bridge iso → **bridge reps** (2 x 8–10 slow reps) *after* your holds.

Day 4: Reintroduce hip control in standing

Today we bias toward standing patterns, because life is standing.

Reset (2 min)

30–60 sec gentle marching in place (low lift)

4 slow breaths

Restore (6–8 min) *(choose 2)*

Supported hip rock-backs (8–10)

90/90 support rotations (6–8/side)

Gentle standing hip extension taps (toe back, small range) 8/side

Reinforce (8–12 min) *(choose 2–3)*

Sit-to-stand (supported as needed)

2–3 x 6–10 reps

Cue: "feet planted, stand tall, no rush."

Split-stance hold (as before)

Side-lying abduction hold or **standing hip abduction (band optional)**

2 x 8–10 slow reps each side

Optional walk: baseline + 0–5 minutes if stable.

Day 5: Consolidate (keep it boring, make it repeatable)

Day 5 is about consistency. Many flare-ups settle when you stop changing the plan daily.

Do Day 4 again with one small quality target:

- no breath holding
- no rushing
- no extra depth hunting

If you feel significantly better, resist the urge to "celebrate" with a big session. Capacity is built by repeatable days, not one victory lap.

Day 6: Gentle single-leg exposure (if tolerated)

Only do this if you can walk without a limp and Day 4–5 were stable.

Add one of the following (pick ONE):

Supported step-up (low step)

2 x 6 each side

Cue: “quiet foot, knee tracks steady, stand tall.”

Single-leg stance with fingertip support

3 x 15–25 sec each side

Cue: “level pelvis, soft knee, breathe.”

Keep everything else the same as Day 4.

If this increases symptoms, remove it and return to Day 4 menu.

Day 7: Review and choose your next phase

Day 7 is a checkpoint, not a test.

Ask three questions:

Is my **baseline** improving? (walking, stairs, sitting tolerance)

- Do symptoms settle within **24 hours** after my plan?
- Do I feel more confident moving?

If yes: you're ready to proceed to **Chapter 6 (Assessment)** and then Phase 1 strength in Chapter 11.
If somewhat: repeat Days 4–6 for another week, making only small progressions.
If no / worsening: review Chapter 3 red flags and consider an assessment.

Step-down rules (if you flare during the week)

A flare-up during a plan doesn't mean failure. It means dose mismatch.

If symptoms spike or you limp:

- Remove the newest addition (usually step-ups or extra walking).
- Cut range by ~25% on mobility drills.

Shift reinforce drills toward **isometrics only** for 48–72 hours.

Keep short, flat walking only if it doesn't worsen next day.

If you cannot bear weight, have severe night pain escalating, systemic signs, or new neurological symptoms, seek care.

Common mistakes (and what to do instead)

Mistake: stretching aggressively because it "feels tight"

Instead: keep mobility gentle and pair it with isometrics. Tightness often softens when the hip feels supported.

Mistake: turning the relief plan into a workout

Instead: this is a nervous-system-friendly week. You're building predictability.

Mistake: adding three progressions at once because you feel better

Instead: change one variable every 48–72 hours.

Mistake: skipping walks entirely

Instead: keep a small baseline walk if tolerated. It's one of the best ways to reintroduce real-world hip load.

Quick checklist / Action plan

- Pick your track (A/B/C) and commit to **7 days** of boring consistency.
- Do **Reset → Restore → Reinforce** daily (15–25 minutes).
- Keep pain 0–3/10 and non-sharp; use the **24-hour check**.
- Progress only one variable at a time, and only when stable.
- If you flare: step down range/volume and return to isometrics for 48–72 hours.

You’re not trying to prove toughness this week. You’re teaching your hip that movement is safe again.

Chapter 6: Hip Mobility Assessment

What this chapter will change for you

- You'll complete a simple, at-home **hip mobility screen** in 8–12 minutes.
- You'll learn what each result likely means for your hip, back, and knee load.
- You'll identify your personal "**limiting direction**" (the motion that needs the most respect and rebuilding).
- You'll leave with a short **mobility prescription** based on your findings, no guesswork.

Why assess at all? Because "tight" is vague

People often say, "My hip is tight." Tight where? In what direction? And does it improve with movement or get worse?

A good assessment does two things:

- shows which motions are currently **limited or sensitive**
- tells you how to train, what to **prioritize**, what to **dose carefully**, and what to **leave alone for now**

This is not a diagnostic test. It's a practical map.

Your assessment rules (keep it safe and useful)

- Warm up with 2–3 minutes of easy walking or gentle marching.
- Move slowly. No bouncing.
- Stay in the **0–3/10** discomfort range, non-sharp.
- Stop if you feel catching, giving way, sharp pain, or a sense of "something's not right."
- Compare sides, but don't obsess, your goal is patterns, not perfection.
- Write down results. Memory lies; notes help.

Scale note: If one test clearly irritates you, skip it and move on. We can still build a plan.

The 6-Test Hip Mobility Screen (8–12 minutes)

Test 1: Comfortable walking check (function first)

How: Walk 30–60 seconds at an easy pace.
Observe:

- Do you limp?
- Is stride shorter on one side?
- Does the foot turn out more on one side?
- Does pain increase or ease as you walk?

What it often means:

- Limp or foot turnout can be a protection strategy. It often shows reduced hip extension/rotation tolerance or hip-abductor fatigue.

- If walking improves symptoms, you're likely dealing with **stiffness + irritability**, not a "do nothing" problem.

Record: limp yes/no, pain location, pain rating, does it warm up?

Test 2: Hip flexion tolerance (knee-to-chest in supine)

How: Lie on your back. Bring one knee toward your chest slowly, stopping before sharp pain or a hard block. Keep the other leg relaxed.
Compare: side to side.

What you're looking for:

- deep groin pinch or sharp front-hip pain
- early stiffness (short of what feels "normal")
- a feeling of blockage vs stretch

What it often means:

- **Front/groin pinch** can indicate hip flexion sensitivity. It doesn't automatically mean "damage," but it does mean you should be conservative with deep squats/lunges for now and earn range gradually.

If it feels more like a stretch in the back of the hip, you may be stiff posteriorly and benefit from gentle flexion work.

Record: range feels limited yes/no, pinch yes/no, discomfort rating.

Test 3: Hip internal rotation (seated 90/90 rotation check)

How: Sit with hips and knees bent about 90°. Keep torso tall. Let one knee gently drop inward (foot moves outward) to test hip **internal rotation**. You can use your hand to guide lightly.
Note: Do not force. Stop at first firm resistance or pain.

What you're looking for:

big side-to-side difference

discomfort deep in hip/groin

early stiffness that makes sitting or squatting feel "blocked"

Why this matters: Internal rotation is a common missing piece in hip pain patterns. When it's limited, the body often borrows rotation from the low back or knee.

What it often means:

- Limited internal rotation + groin discomfort can be a sign you should prioritize **gentle rotation mobility** and avoid deep loaded twisting for now.

- Limited internal rotation without pain often improves with consistent mobility + strength.

Record: "IR limited" mild/moderate/major, pain yes/no.

Test 4: Hip external rotation (figure-4 / seated ankle-on-knee)

How (option A): Sit and place ankle over opposite knee (figure-4).
How (option B): On your back, cross ankle over opposite knee and gently pull thigh in.

What you're looking for:

- buttock stretch vs lateral hip pain

- sharp pinch in groin (less common here)

big asymmetry that matches your symptoms

What it often means:

Lateral hip pain here can suggest abductor or bursa sensitivity, dose carefully with side-lying work and long walks on cambers.

A simple stretch sensation is fine; don't chase intensity.

Record: stretch vs pain, side-to-side difference.

Test 5: Hip extension check (standing stride / "back step" test)

How: Stand tall, hold a wall for balance. Step one foot back as if beginning a lunge, keeping torso upright and pelvis level. Stop when you feel the front of the hip tighten or pain appears.
Key: This is not a deep lunge, just a back-step.

What you're looking for:

front-of-hip tightness that feels "grippy"

pinching

low back arching to compensate

What it often means:

If you can't step back without arching your back, your body is borrowing extension from your spine. This is a common back/hip link.

Front hip "grip" can be hip flexor irritation or protective tone. The answer is usually not aggressive stretching, more often it's controlled extension exposure + glute support (Ch.7–8).

Record: back-step feels restricted yes/no, back arch compensation yes/no, discomfort rating.

Test 6: Single-leg control snapshot (supported single-leg stance)

Mobility isn't just range. It's control.

How: Stand near a counter. Light fingertip support. Lift one foot slightly and hold 15–25 seconds.
Observe:

Does the pelvis drop or hike?

Does the knee cave in?

Do you grip the foot?

Does pain appear quickly?

What it often means:

Quick fatigue or wobble suggests a capacity gap in hip abductors/deep stabilizers. This is one of the strongest predictors of how the hip loads during walking, stairs, and running.

If pain appears quickly, prioritize isometrics and Phase 1 stability before single-leg volume.

Record: time held, pain yes/no, shakiness mild/moderate/high.

Interpreting your results: find your “limiting direction”

Most people have one direction that stands out. Pick the biggest limiter from below:

Limiter A: Flexion-sensitive (knee-to-chest pinch or deep squat pinch)

Common feel: groin pinch, blocked depth, discomfort with sitting low, cycling hard, deep squats.
Focus: reduce deep flexion load temporarily, build strength in tolerable ranges, restore rotation gently.

Limiter B: Rotation-limited (especially internal rotation)

Common feel: stiffness turning, discomfort rolling in bed, back or knee taking rotation load.
Focus: gentle rotation mobility + single-leg control. Rotation often improves when the hip gets stronger and calmer.

Limiter C: Extension-limited (front hip grip, short stride, back arching)

Common feel: tight front hip after sitting, discomfort on hills, back tightness during walking/running.
Focus: extension exposure in small range + glute activation without back compensation.

Limiter D: Control-limited (single-leg stance shaky/painful)

Common feel: pain with stairs, standing on one leg, running fatigue, lateral hip ache after walking.

Focus: Phase 1 stability and progressive single-leg work.

You can have more than one. Choose the top two and keep the plan simple.

Your mobility prescription (based on your limiter)

Do these **5–8 minutes daily** for 2 weeks, then reassess.

If you're Flexion-sensitive

Supported hip rock-backs: 2 x 8 (stop before pinch)

Gentle 90/90 rotations with hands: 2 x 6 each side

Glute bridge iso: 3 x 20 sec (reduce hamstring cramp by bringing feet closer)

If you're Rotation-limited

Seated IR/ER gentle rotations: 2 x 6 each direction

90/90 supported switches: 2 x 6 each side

Split-stance hold: 3 x 20 sec each side (pelvis level)

If you're Extension-limited

Standing back-step (small range): 2 x 6 each side

Standing hip extension taps: 2 x 8 each side

Bridge iso or wall-supported hinge hold: 3 x 20 sec

If you're Control-limited

Supported single-leg stance: 3 x 15–25 sec each side

Side-lying abduction hold (small lift): 2 x 15–20 sec

Sit-to-stand: 2 x 6–8 (slow)

Rule: If a drill reliably increases symptoms next day, reduce range first, then volume.

Common mistakes (and smarter alternatives)

Mistake: Treating the assessment like a stretch contest

Instead: The goal is information. Stop early, stay calm, take notes.

Mistake: Forcing the "tight side" to match the other side immediately

Instead: Aim for gradual change over weeks. Forcing range often increases guarding.

Mistake: Ignoring control because you're focused on mobility

Instead: A hip with less mobility but strong control often functions better than a flexible hip with poor control. Train both.

Quick checklist / Action plan

Complete the 6 tests and write down what you noticed.

Identify your top limiter (and optional second limiter).

Do your matched 5–8 minute mobility prescription daily for 2 weeks.

Reassess after 2 weeks: are you less sensitive, less stiff, more stable?

Move on to Chapter 7 to build glute activation without compensation.

Chapter 7: Glute Activation Without Compensation

What this chapter will change for you

- You'll learn how to "find" your glutes without your low back, hamstrings, or hip flexors stealing the work.
- You'll get a clear activation ladder: **reset → recruit → reinforce → integrate**.
- You'll know the most common compensation patterns (and the exact cues to fix them).
- You'll build a small, repeatable glute routine that supports hip pain relief and protects your knees/back.

Why glutes matter (and why "squeezing" isn't the answer)

Your glutes are not just "power muscles." They're load managers. They help:

- control pelvis position in single-leg stance
- reduce excessive hip drop/rotation during walking and stairs
- distribute force so the front of the hip (flexors) and outer hip tissues don't get overloaded
- keep the knee from doing the hip's job

When glutes aren't contributing well, people often compensate by:

- arching the low back (using spinal extensors)
- gripping hamstrings
- tensing hip flexors
- rotating feet out and "hanging" on ligaments

This isn't weakness as a personal failing. It's coordination. And coordination is trainable.

The goal is not to "turn on" glutes once. The goal is to build glute contribution that shows up during **walking, stairs, squats, and running**, without forcing it.

The glute activation ladder (use this structure)

You'll progress through four steps. If you can't feel glutes in a drill, you don't add complexity, you step back.

Reset: reduce guarding and rib flare

Recruit: get a clean glute contraction in a simple position

Reinforce: add time under tension or reps while keeping it clean

Integrate: bring glutes into standing and single-leg tasks

You'll use this ladder for the rest of the book.

Step 1: Reset - put your trunk in a position your glutes can work from

Most glute "failure" is trunk position failure. If ribs flare up and pelvis tips forward, your back and hip flexors dominate.

Quick reset (60–90 seconds)

90/90 breathing on floor (no equipment)

Lie on your back, knees bent, feet on floor.

Exhale slowly as if fogging a mirror, feel ribs soften down.

On the exhale, gently tuck tailbone 5–10% (not a hard flatten).

Take 4–5 slow breaths.

What you're aiming for:

abdominal wall gently engaged

lower back not aggressively arched

pelvis feels "stacked" under ribs

This isn't core training. It's position training.

Step 2: Recruit - clean glute work in low-threat positions

A) Bridge "set and hold" (the glute finder)

How:

Lie on back, knees bent. Feet hip-width.

Exhale, soften ribs down.

Press through heels and lift hips only to a height where you don't arch your back.

Hold 15–30 seconds.

2–4 sets with 30–45 seconds rest.

Clean cues:

"Ribs down, belt buckle toward chin, just slightly."

"Lift with hips, not with back."

"Heels heavy, toes relaxed."

Common steals (and fixes):

Hamstrings cramp: bring feet *slightly closer* to glutes; lower the lift height; think "push floor away."

Low back tight: reduce height; exhale before lifting; keep ribs down.

Front hip pinch: reduce height; widen stance slightly; try glute squeeze without lifting first.

Regression: glute squeeze holds without lifting: 5 x 10-second squeezes.
Progression: add a mini band above knees and gently press knees out (5–10% effort only).

B) Side-lying abduction hold (glute med, not hip hike)

This targets the lateral glutes that stabilize pelvis and control knee drift.

How:

Lie on side, bottom knee bent, top leg straight.

Slightly roll your top hip forward (so toes point slightly down).

Lift top leg 10–20 cm (small lift).

Hold 15–25 seconds.

2–3 sets each side.

Clean cues:

"Toe slightly down."

"Long leg, quiet waist."

"Do not hike your hip to lift higher."

Steals:

Hip hiking (using QL/side waist): reduce lift height; imagine lengthening your waist.

Hip flexor burn: bring the leg slightly behind midline; reduce lift.

Regression: clam shells with small range (if abduction irritates).
Progression: add a mini band at knees or ankles (only if clean).

C) Prone heel press (glute without back extension)

Great if bridges bother the front of the hip.

How:

Lie face down, forehead on hands.

Bend one knee to 90°.

Gently press the heel toward the ceiling *without* lifting your pelvis or arching your back.

Hold 10–20 seconds.

3 sets each side.

Cue: "Heel up, pelvis heavy."
If your low back tightens, reduce intensity to 30–50% effort.

Step 3: Reinforce - build endurance before power

For hip pain, endurance usually matters more than max strength early on. Your hip needs glutes to show up for many reps: walking steps, stair climbs, runs.

The "2+1" template (simple and repeatable)

Do this 3–5 days/week for two weeks:

Bridge hold: **3 x 20–30 sec**

Side-lying abduction hold: **2–3 x 15–25 sec/side**
+1 optional: prone heel press **2 x 15 sec/side**

Rule: keep it clean. If compensation appears, stop the set early. Quality builds capacity faster than pushing sloppy volume.

Step 4: Integrate - glutes in standing (where life happens)

Activation drills are only useful if they carry over. Integration is where you teach the glutes to contribute while you stand, step, and shift.

A) Hip hinge to wall (glute loading without back strain)

How:

Stand about 20–30 cm from a wall, facing away from it.

Slightly bend knees, keep ribs stacked.

Push hips back to tap the wall, then return tall.

2 x 8–10 slow reps.

Cue: "Hips back, shins mostly vertical, chest quiet."
If your back arches, reduce range.

B) Supported split-stance hold (glute + pelvis control)

How:

One foot forward, one back, light hand support.

Keep pelvis level (no hip drop).

Hold 20–30 seconds each side.

2–3 sets.

What this trains: the glute's real job, single-leg-ish stability without the demand of full single-leg stance.

Cue: "Front heel heavy, zipper up through the center."
If front knee caves, reduce stance length and focus on gentle knee tracking.

C) Lateral wall press (glute med "switch on" in standing)

How:

Stand side-on to a wall. Knee slightly bent.

Press the outside of your knee or thigh gently into the wall (20–40% effort).

Hold 15–25 seconds.

2–3 sets each side.

Cue: "Press and breathe, don't lean your whole body." You should feel lateral glute, not low back.

The compensation map (so you can self-correct fast)

Compensation 1: Low back takeover

Looks like: rib flare, big arch, feeling it in lumbar spine. **Fix:** exhale first; reduce range; keep lift lower; think "ribs down, pelvis heavy."

Compensation 2: Hamstring dominance

Looks like: cramps, hamstring burn, glutes feel absent.
Fix: feet slightly closer; push through heels; lower lift height; shorten holds.

Compensation 3: Hip flexor gripping

Looks like: front hip pinch/burn, especially in bridges or standing drills.
Fix: reduce hip flexion depth elsewhere; keep drills small; add prone heel press; avoid forcing hip extension stretches.

Compensation 4: Hip hiking / side waist dominance

Looks like: you lift the pelvis instead of lifting the leg (side-lying work), or you lean in standing.
Fix: smaller range; "long waist"; use wall press with breath.

Common mistakes (and better moves)

Mistake: Searching for a massive burn

Instead: seek a steady, local effort you can repeat. Glutes respond to consistency more than drama.

Mistake: Doing advanced band walks when you can't control pelvis

Instead: earn it with holds and split-stance control first.

Mistake: Over-bracing your core

Instead: gentle stacking, steady breathing. You want support, not rigidity.

Mistake: Training glutes but ignoring walking mechanics

Instead: glute work is preparation. Walking (Chapter 10) is practice.

Quick checklist / Action plan

Do the 60–90 second reset before glute drills.

Choose **two recruit drills** (bridge hold + side-lying hold is a great start).

Train 3–5 days/week for 2 weeks using the "2+1" template.

- Stop sets before compensation appears; quality is the progression.
- If front hip irritation increases, reduce bridge height and add prone heel presses.

Glutes don't need to be "on" all day. They need to show up at the right time, at the right dose, in the right tasks. That's exactly what you're building.

Chapter 8: Hip Flexors: Tight vs Irritated

What this chapter will change for you

You'll learn how to tell the difference between hip flexors that feel "tight" versus hip flexors that are **irritated and protective**.

You'll stop defaulting to aggressive stretching and instead use a safer **calm-and-load** approach.

You'll get a flexor-friendly progression: **settle → support → strengthen → reintroduce extension**.

You'll know when front-of-hip pain is more likely coming from the hip joint, the flexors, or compensation patterns.

Why hip flexors get blamed for everything

Hip flexors sit at the front of the hip. When you sit, climb stairs, sprint, or lift your knee, they're involved. When the hip is irritated, many people feel discomfort in the same region, front hip/groin, so the flexors get blamed automatically.

Sometimes that's correct. Sometimes it isn't.

The key is this: **"tight" is a sensation, not a diagnosis.** Tightness can be:

- normal stiffness from sitting
- protective tone due to irritation
- weakness/fatigue (a muscle that's working too hard feels tight)
- a strategy to stabilize a hip that doesn't feel stable
- sensitivity from the joint or nearby tissues

Your job isn't to guess perfectly. Your job is to respond intelligently and safely.

Tight vs irritated: the simplest practical difference

Use this quick decision test:

It's more likely "tight/stiff" if:

- it feels better after gentle movement or heat

- stretching feels relieving and doesn't worsen symptoms next day
- discomfort is mild and diffuse (not sharp)
- you can load it lightly without a sharp response

It's more likely "irritated/protective" if:

- deep stretching increases pain for hours or next day
- you feel pinching, catching, or sharp discomfort at the front/groin
- it flares with hills, stairs, long strides, or long sitting then sudden activity
- it makes you shorten your stride or avoid hip extension
- you feel tenderness near the front of the hip and it's reactive

Translation: If stretching reliably makes it worse, stop forcing range. Switch to calm loading.

A note on "pinching" in the front of the hip

Front-of-hip pinching is common. It can reflect hip flexion sensitivity, joint irritation, or poor control in deep flexion. It can also happen if you're trying to stretch into extension aggressively while the hip is already protective.

What matters most is not the label, it's your response:

reduce the aggravating depth/position temporarily

build strength and control in tolerable ranges

reintroduce extension gradually, not heroically

The practical system: Settle → Support → Strengthen → Reintroduce

Step 1: Settle (reduce threat and tone)

If your front hip feels "grippy," start here for 3–7 days.

A) 90/90 breathing reset (2 minutes)
Same as Chapter 7. Soft ribs down, gentle pelvic stacking.

B) Gentle marching (1 minute)
Small knee lifts, slow, pain-free. This is a "keep it safe" signal to the flexors.

C) Short-range hip flexor isometric (optional, if tolerated)

Stand holding a counter

Lift knee slightly (10–20 cm)

Hold 10–20 seconds, 2–3 reps each side
Intensity should be 30–50% effort.

Why: Isometrics can reduce pain sensitivity while maintaining muscle engagement, without forcing range.

Step 2: Support (teach the hip to extend without borrowing from the back)

Often the hip flexors feel tight because the hip doesn't extend well, so the back tries to do it. Your flexors then guard more.

Standing back-step (small range)

Hold a wall for support

Step one foot back slightly, stay tall

Stop before pinching or back arching

2 x 6 reps each side

Key cue: "Tailbone heavy, ribs quiet."
If you feel it in the low back, reduce range and slow down.

Step 3: Strengthen (build flexor capacity instead of stretching it endlessly)

Many "tight" flexors are actually under-conditioned for the demands placed on them (stairs, running, standing from chairs, long walking). Strengthen them gently.

Option A: Supine bent-knee march (low threat)

Lie on back, knees bent

Exhale gently, ribs down

Lift one foot a few centimeters, then lower

2–3 x 8 slow reps each side

Cue: “Quiet pelvis. Small lift.”

Option B: Seated knee lift isometrics (very controlled)

Sit tall on a chair

Lift one knee slightly and hold 10–20 seconds

2–3 holds each side

Progression: add a light band around feet or a small ankle weight later, but only if symptoms stay stable.

Option C: Standing band march (later in the program)

We’ll use this as you enter Phase 2/3, when single-leg control is stronger.

Step 4: Reintroduce extension (earn length safely)

Stretching is not banned. It just needs the right timing and dosage.

Use this guideline: **Do extension exposure after you've supported and strengthened**, and keep it gentle.

Gentle hip flexor "open" (not a deep lunge stretch)

Half-kneeling or standing split stance with support

Tuck pelvis slightly (5–10%), ribs down

Shift forward a few centimeters

Hold 15–25 seconds, 1–2 rounds each side

Stop if: pinching, sharp pain, or symptoms worsen later that day.

Better metric than "deep stretch": you can walk with a longer stride comfortably.

Common front-hip scenarios (and what to do)

Scenario 1: "It feels tight after sitting"

Likely: stiffness + reduced extension practice
Do: movement interrupts + gentle back-step + bridge

holds
Avoid: long aggressive stretching as your main strategy

Scenario 2: "It burns on hills or stairs"

Likely: flexors doing too much because glutes aren't sharing load
Do: glute routine (Ch.7) + short-range flexor strengthening + reduce hill volume temporarily

Scenario 3: "Pinching in deep squats/lunges"

Likely: flexion sensitivity + control deficit in deep range
Do: reduce depth, strengthen through tolerable range, build single-leg control, then earn depth back later
Avoid: forcing depth with heavy load

Scenario 4: "Front hip pain during bridges"

Likely: extension strategy issue or anterior hip sensitivity
Do: lower bridge height, widen stance slightly, try prone heel press instead, keep ribs stacked

---

Common mistakes (and steadier alternatives)

Mistake: Treating hip flexors like a tight rubber band

Instead: treat them like a load-bearing tissue that needs the right dose of strength and motion.

Mistake: Stretching harder when the hip is already irritated

Instead: settle with isometrics and short-range control for 3–7 days, then reintroduce gentle extension.

Mistake: Ignoring the trunk position

Instead: stack ribs over pelvis. A calm trunk gives the flexors a safer environment.

Mistake: Returning to hills/sprints too soon

Instead: rebuild baseline walking first, then reintroduce hills with progression rules.

Quick checklist / Action plan

Decide: does stretching help (tight) or worsen (irritated)?

If irritated: use **Settle + Support** for 3–7 days (breathing, small marches, back-steps).

Add flexor strengthening 2–4 days/week (supine marches or seated isometrics).

Reintroduce gentle extension holds only if symptoms remain stable over 24 hours.

Track success by function: longer stride, easier stairs, less front-hip grip.

Hip flexors don't need to be "loosened into submission." They need a calmer environment and a smarter workload.

Chapter 9: Adductors and Pelvic Stability

What this chapter will change for you

You'll understand why inner-thigh (adductor) capacity is a major part of **hip and pelvic stability**, not an afterthought.

You'll learn to spot when adductors are **overworking** versus when they're **undertrained**.

You'll get a safe progression to rebuild adductor strength without provoking groin pain: **support → isometrics → controlled range → integration**.

You'll reduce the "wobble" that often shows up as hip pain, back tightness, or knee irritation during single-leg tasks.

Why adductors matter more than you've been told

Adductors (inner-thigh muscles) don't just pull the leg inward. They help:

- stabilize the pelvis when you're on one leg (walking, stairs)
- control hip position during squats, lunges, and direction changes
- share load with glutes and deep hip rotators
- support the hip joint in deeper ranges (especially flexion + rotation)

If adductors are weak or easily irritated, the body often compensates by:

- gripping hip flexors
- leaning the trunk
- overusing the outer hip tissues (lateral hip soreness)
- letting the knee drift inward during single-leg tasks

That's why adductor capacity is a quiet "missing link" in many hip pain plans.

Two common adductor patterns (so you don't treat the wrong problem)

Pattern A: The "overworking adductor"

Often shows up as:

- inner groin tightness after walking/running
- discomfort during side steps, lateral lunges, quick direction changes
- pain that spikes with sudden increases in training volume
- tenderness high in the inner thigh

What's usually happening: the adductors are trying to stabilize a pelvis that doesn't feel secure, often because glutes/core stacking aren't sharing the job yet.

Pattern B: The "undertrained adductor"

Often shows up as:

- wobble/instability in single-leg stance
- knee collapse during stairs or lunges
- discomfort in deep squat positions or coming out of the bottom
- chronic groin sensitivity with predictable loading

What's usually happening: the adductors don't have enough capacity for real-life tasks, so they flare when asked.

Both patterns benefit from training, but the **dose** and **starting position** matter.

The pelvis concept: "level enough" and "quiet enough"

Pelvic stability is not rigid stillness. It's the ability to keep your pelvis **level enough** and **quiet enough** while you move.

Think of your pelvis like a bowl of water. You don't need it perfectly still. You just don't want it sloshing wildly with every step.

Adductors help prevent the pelvis from drifting and twisting excessively, especially when the hip is flexed and loaded (stairs, running, squats). When adductors do their job, the hip feels less "pinchy" and the knee tracks more steadily.

The practical system: Support → Isometrics → Controlled range → Integration

Step 1: Support (reduce groin threat)

If you have groin sensitivity, start with positions that feel safe.

Support principles:

- smaller ranges
- shorter lever arms (bent knee instead of straight)
- lower intensity (30–60%)
- steady breathing (no bracing battles)

Step 2: Isometrics (the safest entry point for most people)

Isometrics are your friend for irritated groin tissues. They tend to be joint-friendly and help build tolerance without provoking big soreness.

A) Pillow squeeze (supine adductor iso)

How:

Lie on your back, knees bent, feet on floor.

Place a pillow or yoga block between knees.

Gently squeeze at 30–50% effort.

Hold 20–30 seconds.

Do: 4–6 holds, resting 20–30 seconds between.

Cues:

"Steady squeeze, no shaking."

"Breathe slowly; don't hold your breath."

"Pelvis stays quiet."

Progression: increase effort to 60–70% as long as symptoms stay stable.

B) Side-lying adductor hold (short lever)

How:

- Lie on your side. Bottom leg straight, top knee bent with foot in front for support.
- Lift the bottom leg slightly (small lift).
- Hold 10–20 seconds.

Do: 2–4 holds each side.

Cue: "Small lift, long leg, quiet trunk."
Regression: skip if it provokes groin pain, use pillow squeezes first.
Progression: longer holds or more reps.

Step 3: Controlled range strength (earn motion under control)

When isometrics are stable for 1–2 weeks, add controlled movement.

A) Standing adductor slide (towel slide)

How:

Stand holding a counter for support.

Place one foot on a towel on a smooth floor.

Slowly slide the foot out to the side a small distance, then back in.

Keep pelvis level; don't lean.

Do: 2–3 x 6–10 each side.

Cue: "Quiet pelvis, smooth slide."
Stop if: sharp groin pain or catching.

B) Supported lateral step (micro side lunge pattern)

This is not a deep side lunge. It's a controlled weight shift.

How:

Take a small step to the side.

Sit hips back slightly (tiny hinge), keep knee tracking, then push back to center.

Use support as needed.

Do: 2 x 6 each side.

Cue: "Small range, hips back, push the floor away."
Progression: gradually increase step width over weeks, not days.

Step 4: Integration (adductors working with glutes in real tasks)

Adductors and glutes are teammates, not rivals.

A) Split-stance adductor bias hold

How:

- Stand in a split stance and shift slightly toward the front leg.
- Gently "hug" the front foot toward the midline (without actually moving it).
- Hold 15–25 seconds.

Do: 2–3 holds each side.

Cue: "Gentle inward intent, pelvis level, breathe."
This builds adductor contribution in a stance you use constantly.

B) **Copenhagen "lite" (only if you're stable)**

This can be excellent but it's easy to overdose, so treat it with respect.

How (lite version):

Side plank from knees (bottom knee on floor).

Top leg rests on a low bench/chair with knee bent.

Lift hips gently and hold 10–15 seconds.

Do: 2–3 holds each side.

Rule: If you get groin soreness that lingers >24 hours, regress to pillow squeezes and slides for two weeks before retrying.

How to choose your starting point

Use your 24-hour response as your guide.

Start with isometrics if:

- groin area is sensitive to stretching or quick movements
- you get sharp discomfort in deeper positions
- you flare with side steps or lateral lunges

Start with controlled range if:

- groin feels stiff but not reactive
- you tolerate walking and stairs well
- pain is more "weakness/effort" than sharpness

Common mistakes (and what to do instead)

Mistake: Deep groin stretching when the adductors are irritated

Instead: isometrics first. Stretching an irritated tissue often increases protection.

Mistake: Jumping straight into big side lunges or heavy Copenhagen work

Instead: earn it with short-lever holds and controlled slides. Adductors respond well to progression, but they punish impatience.

Mistake: Letting the pelvis drift and calling it "strength"

Instead: keep the pelvis "level enough." If you have to lean, the set is too hard.

Mistake: Only training outer hip muscles

Instead: balance the system. Outer hip strength without inner hip capacity can still leave you unstable in single-leg tasks.

Quick checklist / Action plan

If you have groin sensitivity: do **pillow squeezes** 4–6 holds, 3–5 days/week for 2 weeks.

Add **standing towel slides** 2–3 days/week once isometrics are stable.

Integrate with split-stance adductor bias holds to teach real-world carryover.

Use the 24-hour check: if next-day symptoms spike, reduce range and intensity before reducing all movement.

Remember the goal: a pelvis that is "quiet enough" during walking, stairs, squats, and running.

Strong adductors don't make you tight. They make you stable, and stability is one of the most reliable ways to calm hip pain.

Chapter 10: Walking Mechanics for Hip Health

What this chapter will change for you

You'll learn how to walk in a way that reduces hip irritation without obsessing over "perfect form."

You'll spot the most common walking compensations (stride shortening, foot turnout, trunk lean) and know what to adjust first.

You'll set a repeatable walking **baseline** and use simple rules to progress volume safely.

You'll build a short "walk prep" routine that improves hip comfort and protects your back and knees.

Why walking is both the test and the tool

Walking is the most common single-leg task you do. It's also the easiest way to accumulate hip load without realizing it. If your hip hurts, walking can feel threatening, but for most non-red-flag cases, **the right dose of walking is medicine**.

The goal isn't to walk "perfectly." The goal is to walk with:

- less protective compensation
- steadier single-leg control
- a dose you can repeat without flare-ups

Walking doesn't just reflect hip health. Done well, it builds it.

The three walking variables that matter most

Forget a long checklist. For hip pain, three variables usually drive comfort:

1) Stride length (often too long or too short)

- If you overstride, you can increase front-hip irritation and joint compression.
- If you understride, you may stiffen the hip and borrow from the back.

Target: a "medium" stride that feels smooth, not forced. Think: shorter than a power walk, longer than a shuffle.

2) Pelvis control (level enough)

A large hip drop or trunk sway can increase lateral hip load and knee stress. But rigidity isn't the goal either.

Target: pelvis stays relatively steady; your trunk doesn't lurch side-to-side.

3) Foot direction (avoid excessive turnout as a default)

Many people turn the foot out to avoid hip rotation demands. Sometimes it's useful temporarily. Long-term, it can keep the hip from regaining options.

Target: feet point mostly forward (not military straight), with a natural slight turnout.

The walking self-check (60 seconds)

Do this on a flat surface.

Step 1: Walk for 20–30 seconds as you normally do. Notice:

- pain location and intensity

any limp

foot turnout

trunk lean

Step 2: Repeat for 20–30 seconds with these three adjustments:

Slightly shorter stride

“Quiet trunk” (imagine your head gliding forward, not swaying)

Soft, steady pace (no rushing)

Step 3: Ask: did it feel better, worse, or the same?

This tells you whether mechanics changes help. If they help, you have a lever.

The “quiet walking” cues (simple, not obsessive)

Use one cue at a time. Over-cueing makes you tense.

Cue A: “Shorter and softer”

Slightly shorten stride and soften the foot contact.

- Helpful for front-of-hip irritation and groin sensitivity.
- Often reduces joint compression spikes.

Cue B: "Push the ground behind you"

Instead of reaching forward with the leg, feel a gentle push behind you.

- Helpful for extension-limited hips and back/hip linkage.
- Encourages glute contribution.

Cue C: "Zip up the zipper"

Imagine a zipper from pubic bone to sternum staying gently lifted and stacked.

- Helpful if you arch your back or sway.

Cue D: "Knees track, don't dive"

If your knee collapses inward as you step, think: knee tracks over mid-foot.

Helpful for knee symptoms and lateral hip overload.

Pick one cue and use it for 1–2 minutes, then let it go. Walking should still feel natural.

Common walking compensations (and what to change first)

Compensation 1: Limping or unloading the painful side

What it does: increases load on the other side and often irritates back/knee.
First change: reduce walking dose and slow pace until you can walk without a limp. If you can't, that's a sign to scale aggressively and consider evaluation (Chapter 3).

Compensation 2: Big trunk lean over the painful hip

This is a common strategy to reduce hip abductor demand.
First change: shorten stride slightly and slow down. Then add lateral hip endurance work (Chapter 7) and split-stance holds.

Compensation 3: Foot turned out a lot ("duck walk")

Often reduces rotation demand at the hip but can increase knee stress or keep the hip stiff.
First change: don't force feet straight. Just reduce turnout by **10–20%** and see if symptoms improve. Pair with rotation mobility (Chapter 6) and single-leg control training.

Compensation 4: Overstriding (reaching forward)

Often increases front hip irritation and can irritate hamstrings and back.
First change: shorten stride and slightly increase cadence (more steps per minute without speed increase).

Walking dosage: baseline, progression, and the flare-proof rules

Walking is one of the easiest ways to overdose because it's "just walking." Treat it like training.

Step 1: Find your baseline

Your baseline is the longest walk you can do that:

- stays within 0–3/10 discomfort
- does not create a limp
- returns you near baseline within 24 hours

If you flare after 30 minutes, start at 10–15. Baseline is about repeatability.

Baseline options:

- 1 walk/day at baseline time
- OR 2 shorter walks/day (often better for irritable hips)

Step 2: Progress with boring consistency

Progress only when stable for 3–5 days.

Choose one progression:

- Add **2–5 minutes** to one walk
- Or add a second short walk
- Or add a small hill dose (only after flat is stable)

Keep increases to **10–20%** max per week. If you're sensitive, use 5–10%.

Step 3: Hills and stairs are multipliers

A 20-minute hilly walk can load the hip like a much longer flat walk.

Rule: don't add hills and distance in the same week. If hills trigger front hip or lateral hip pain, keep them minimal until Phase 1 strength is consistent.

Step 4: The 24-hour walking check

- If next day is worse: reduce time by 20–30% and stay flat.
- If two days in a row are worse: step back further and prioritize the 7-day plan menu for 3–5 days.

Your walk-prep routine (3–5 minutes)

Do this before walks if you're stiff, or after sitting.

- **Standing weight shifts**: 30 seconds

Supported hip hinge to wall: 8 reps

Back-step taps (small range): 6 each side

Supported single-leg stance: 15 seconds each side

This is not warm-up theater. It's a quick signal: "hips online."

Troubleshooting: three common situations

"My hip hurts more at the start, then eases"

Often stiffness + protective tone.
Do: walk 2–3 minutes, then pause for 30 seconds of weight shifts, then continue. Consider two shorter walks.

"My hip is fine during the walk, worse later"

Often dose is too high, or hills/pace are too aggressive.
Do: reduce time by 20–30%, slow down, and keep cadence slightly higher (shorter steps).

"My knee starts aching when I fix my hip"

Common when you change mechanics too abruptly.
Do: make smaller changes (10–20% adjustments), and prioritize hip strength phases so the system can support the new pattern.

Quick checklist / Action plan

- Set a walking baseline you can repeat without limping or next-day worsening.

- Use one cue at a time: **shorter/softer**, **push behind**, **quiet trunk**, or **knee tracks**.

- Progress walking only after 3–5 stable days, and by 10–20% max per week (less if sensitive).

- Treat hills and stairs as load multipliers, add them slowly.

- Use the 3–5 minute walk-prep routine on stiff days.

Walking shouldn't feel like a test you might fail. It's one of your most reliable tools to rebuild hip confidence, when you dose it like training.

Chapter 11: Strength Phase 1: Foundational Stability

What this chapter will change for you

You'll build a Phase 1 strength base that makes daily movement feel safer: **stairs, standing, walking, getting up/down**.

You'll learn how to train hip strength without provoking flare-ups: **low threat, high consistency**

You'll get a Phase 1 menu with clear **regressions/progressions** and simple weekly structure.

You'll use decision rules to know exactly when to **progress, hold, or step back**.

What "foundational stability" actually means

Phase 1 is not about lifting heavy. It's about teaching your hip to accept and transfer load without panicking.

Foundational stability includes:

- **stacking**: ribs over pelvis so your hip muscles aren't fighting your posture
- **control**: the pelvis stays "quiet enough" during basic tasks
- **tolerance**: tissues handle repeated loading without next-day spikes
- **capacity**: you can do the basics (walk, stairs, sit-to-stand) more easily

If Phase 1 is done well, Phase 2 feels like a natural next step, not a leap.

The Phase 1 priorities (in order)

- **Pain-sensitive tissues calm down** through smart dosing
- **Glute + adductor support** increases (Ch.7–9)
- **Trunk and pelvis** coordinate under load
- **Basic patterns** (hinge, squat-to-chair, split stance) become steady

This is "quiet competence." That's the base.

Your Phase 1 rules (the ones that prevent setbacks)

- Train 2–4 days/week depending on irritability.
- Keep discomfort **0–3/10**, non-sharp.
- Stop sets before compensation takes over (limp, knee collapse, trunk lurch).
- Use the **24-hour check**. If worse tomorrow, reduce range/volume next time.
- Progress only one variable at a time, and only after **3–5 stable days**.

The Phase 1 Menu (choose 5–6 exercises per session)

Category A: Hip-friendly squat pattern

1) Sit-to-stand (chair squat)

3 x 6–10 reps

Start from a chair height that feels safe.

Cues: "Feet heavy, stand tall, slow down on the way down."
Regression: higher chair or hands on thighs.
Progression: lower chair, slower tempo (3 seconds down), light weight held at chest.

Category B: Hinge pattern (hip load without deep flexion)

2) Hip hinge to wall

2–3 x 8–12 reps

Cues: "Hips back, ribs quiet, shins mostly vertical."
Regression: smaller range.
Progression: hold a backpack or dumbbell (light), or add a 2-second pause at the wall.

Category C: Split-stance stability (halfway to single-leg)

3) Supported split-stance hold

3 x 20–30 sec each side

Cues: "Front heel heavy, pelvis level, breathe."
Regression: shorter stance and more hand support.
Progression: reduce hand support, increase hold time to 40 sec, or add a very small bend-and-rise (mini split squat) 2 x 6.

Category D: Lateral hip stability (glute med endurance)

4) Lateral wall press hold

2–3 x 15–25 sec each side

Cues: "Press gently, don't lean."
Regression: lower effort (20–30%).
Progression: longer holds or add a small single-leg stance component (stand on outside leg, press inside leg into wall lightly).

Category E: Adductor support (pelvic stability partner)

5) Pillow squeeze isometric

4–6 x 20–30 sec

Cues: "Steady squeeze, breathe, pelvis quiet."
Regression: reduce effort to 20–30%.
Progression: increase effort to 60–70% or switch to towel slides (Ch.9) 2 x 6–10.

Category F: Posterior chain support (glutes without back takeover)

6) Bridge hold or bridge reps

Holds: 3 x 20–30 sec

OR reps: 2–3 x 8–12 slow reps

Cues: "Ribs down, lift to your safe height."
Regression: smaller lift or glute squeezes only.
Progression: mini band above knees (light), or single-leg bridge **only later** (Phase 2).

Category G: Calf/foot tolerance (often overlooked)

Your hip and knee load depend on what the foot/calf can handle.

7) Calf raise (supported)

2–3 x 10–15 reps

Cues: "Slow up, slow down, don't roll ankles."
Regression: two-leg only, small range.
Progression: single-leg supported calf raises.

Category H: Optional gentle step (only if walking is stable)

8) Low step-up (supported)

2 x 6–8 each side

Cues: "Quiet foot, knee steady, stand tall."
Regression: smaller step or reduce reps.
Progression: add a pause at the top (1–2 seconds).

Rule: If step-ups trigger lateral hip pain or groin pinch, pause them and build more capacity with split stance and sit-to-stand first.

Two simple Phase 1 workouts (rotate them)

Do A and B on alternating days.

Workout A (30–35 minutes)

Sit-to-stand: 3 x 6–10

Hinge to wall: 2–3 x 8–12

Split-stance holds: 3 x 20–30 sec/side

Lateral wall press: 2–3 x 15–25 sec/side

Bridge holds: 3 x 20–30 sec

Optional calf raises: 2 x 12–15

Workout B (25–35 minutes)

Sit-to-stand (slower): 3 x 6–8

Pillow squeeze: 4–6 x 20 sec

Split-stance mini bends: 2 x 6/side (or holds if sensitive)

- Side-lying abduction holds (from Ch.7): 2 x 15–25 sec/side
- Hinge to wall: 2 x 10
- Optional low step-ups: 2 x 6/side

Frequency:

- High irritability: 2 days/week + daily short mobility
- Moderate: 3 days/week
- Low: 4 days/week (but keep sessions moderate)

Progressions: how to know when Phase 1 is "done enough"

You're ready for Phase 2 when most of these are true:

- You can walk your baseline without limping and without next-day worsening
- Sit-to-stand feels smoother and less painful

Split-stance holds feel steady (minimal wobble)

Lateral wall press holds feel strong and non-irritating

You can do a low step-up without compensation or flare-ups

Pain is stable and predictable, not “spiky”

Phase 1 is usually **2–4 weeks**, sometimes longer if symptoms are sensitive. Longer is not failure, longer is often smarter.

Common mistakes (and what to do instead)

Mistake: Going heavy too soon because Phase 1 feels “too easy”

Instead: treat Phase 1 like joint insurance. The goal is repeatability and control, not fatigue.

Mistake: Deep ranges before you’ve earned them

Instead: use comfortable ranges now; depth returns later through capacity, not forcing.

Mistake: Training to the point your form collapses

Instead: stop sets early. Compensation is your "stop sign," not a challenge.

Mistake: Skipping rest days when tissues are irritable

Instead: strength days 2–4/week, mobility most days, walking baseline daily if tolerated.

Quick checklist / Action plan

Choose 2–4 strength days/week based on irritability.

Use Workout A/B rotation and keep discomfort 0–3/10.

Progress one variable at a time after 3–5 stable days.

If next day is worse: reduce range first, then volume, then load.

Move to Phase 2 only when walking and split-stance control are steady.

Phase 1 isn't glamorous. It's the foundation that makes everything else feel safer, and that's exactly why it works.

Chapter 12: Strength Phase 2: Single-Leg Control

What this chapter will change for you

- You'll build the kind of hip strength that actually shows up in life: **stairs, walking speed, uneven ground, running prep**.
- You'll learn to train single-leg work without triggering flare-ups by using the right "bridge" exercises.
- You'll get a Phase 2 progression that improves pelvis control, knee tracking, and hip confidence.
- You'll know exactly when to progress, and how to step back without losing momentum.

Why single-leg control is the hinge point

Most hip pain persists because daily life is a repeated single-leg task. Every step is a small single-leg squat. Every stair is a bigger one. If your hip can't control load on one leg, the system solves it with compensation: trunk lean, foot turnout, knee collapse, back stiffness, or overuse of outer hip tissues.

Single-leg control is not about balancing like a gymnast. It's about three quiet skills:

- **Load acceptance** (you can take bodyweight without flinching)
- **Pelvis steadiness** (no big drop/hike)
- **Knee tracking** (not rigid, not collapsing)

Phase 2 teaches those skills with progressive exposure.

The Phase 2 prerequisites (don't skip these)

You're ready for Phase 2 when:

- you can walk your baseline without limping and without next-day worsening
- split-stance holds feel steady (Phase 1)
- sit-to-stand is controlled through a comfortable range
- your lateral hip work (wall press or side-lying holds) doesn't flare symptoms

If you're not there yet, Phase 2 will feel like a fight. Staying in Phase 1 a little longer is not "behind." It's intelligent pacing.

The Phase 2 principles (how we make it safe)

- **Support first:** use a wall/counter until control improves.
- **Short ranges first:** earn depth slowly.
- **Slow tempo:** speed hides compensation.
- **Fewer reps, better reps:** stop before quality drops.
- **One new stress at a time:** don't add running, hills, and single-leg strength all in the same week.

The Phase 2 Menu (choose 5–7 per session)

Category A: Single-leg stance skill (the base layer)

1) Supported single-leg stance

3 x 20–40 sec each side

Fingertips on counter; reduce support gradually.

Cues: "Soft knee, level pelvis, breathe."
Regression: toe-touch stance (back toe lightly on floor).
Progression: eyes forward, less hand support, small head turns.

Category B: Step pattern (stairs practice with control)

2) Step-up + controlled lower (eccentric focus)

2–3 x 6–8 each side

Use a low step initially.

Cues:

"Quiet foot."

"Knee tracks over mid-foot."

"Lower slowly, own the descent."

Regression: smaller step; use more hand support; reduce reps.
Progression: slightly higher step, pause at top, or slower lowering (3 seconds down).

Category C: Single-leg squat pattern (scaled)

3) Supported split squat (shallow range)

2–3 x 6–10 each side

Hold support and keep range modest.

Cues: "Drop straight down, stay tall, front heel heavy."
Regression: split-stance holds only.
Progression: deeper range, less support, add light load later.

Category D: Hip hinge single-leg bridge (without full single-leg bridge yet)

4) Kickstand RDL (hinge with one leg assisting)

2–3 x 6–10 each side

Back foot is a "kickstand" for balance; most load on front leg.

Cues: "Hips back, spine quiet, weight through mid-foot/heel."
Regression: two-leg hinge.
Progression: hold weight (light), increase hinge depth gradually.

Category E: Lateral control (hip abductors under load)

5) Lateral step-down (very small range)

Stand on a step; tap the opposite heel to the floor lightly.

2 x 5–8 each side.

Cues: “Pelvis level, knee tracks, control the down.”
Regression: do it from a book/very low step or do supported single-leg stance instead.
Progression: increase step height slowly or add reps.

Note: If lateral hip pain flares here, it’s often too much too soon, go back to wall press + step-ups.

Category F: Adductor + pelvis integration

6) Standing towel slide (adductor control)

2–3 x 6–10 each side

Cues: “Smooth slide, quiet pelvis, don’t lean.”
Progression: slightly wider slide or add a brief pause.

Category G: Glute integration (dynamic, not just holds)

7) Lateral band walk (only if clean)

Mini band above knees or at ankles (light).

2 x 8–12 steps each direction.

Cues: "Small steps, knees track, pelvis quiet."
Regression: wall press holds.
Progression: more steps or slightly stronger band, only if no next-day flare.

Two Phase 2 workouts (rotate)

Workout A (30–40 minutes)

Supported single-leg stance: 3 x 20–40 sec/side

Step-up + slow lower: 3 x 6/side

Supported split squat: 2–3 x 6–10/side

Kickstand RDL: 2–3 x 6–10/side

Wall press hold or band walk: 2 sets

Optional calf raises: 2 x 12–15

Workout B (30–40 minutes)

Toe-touch single-leg stance: 3 x 30 sec/side

Lateral step-down (small): 2 x 5–8/side

- Step-up (slightly higher or pause): 2 x 6–8/side
- Towel slides: 2 x 8/side
- Bridge reps (if tolerated): 2 x 10–12
- Side-lying abduction holds: 2 x 15–20 sec/side

Frequency: 2–4 days/week depending on irritability and recovery.

Progression targets (how you know you're building real control)

You should notice:

- stairs feel steadier and less "grabby" in the hip
- you can stand on one leg with less wobble
- knee tracks more reliably (less diving inward)
- walking pace improves without pain spikes
- lateral hip soreness decreases over time

These are the markers that Phase 2 is doing its job.

Decision rules: when to move forward

Progress when:

- you can complete a session with no limping
- next day symptoms are near baseline
- you feel stable, not "held together" by tension
- you've had 3–5 stable days

Progress by changing **one** variable:

- add 1 set, OR
- add 2 reps, OR
- increase step height slightly, OR
- reduce hand support, OR
- add a small load to kickstand RDL

Hold when:

- symptoms fluctuate but don't worsen
- sleep/stress is high
- a new exercise still feels "novel"

Step back when:

- pain spikes >5/10 during training
- lateral hip pain escalates after step-downs/band walks
- next day is clearly worse or you develop a limp

Step back by reducing range or removing the most provocative drill (often step-downs/band walks) for 1–2 weeks while maintaining the rest.

Common mistakes (and what to do instead)

Mistake: Going full single-leg too soon

Instead: kickstand variations and support are the bridge. Earn independence.

Mistake: Letting the knee collapse and calling it "strength"

Instead: reduce range and use support. Knee tracking is a quality marker, not a bonus.

Mistake: Turning Phase 2 into high-rep burnout

Instead: keep reps moderate. Stop sets when control fades. Endurance will build through consistency.

Mistake: Adding running at the same time as Phase 2 progressions

Instead: if you're returning to running, keep strength stable and progress running conservatively (Chapter 15).

Quick checklist / Action plan

- Use support and shallow ranges first, make it clean before making it hard.

- Train 2–4 days/week using the A/B workouts.
- Prioritize step-ups, split squats, kickstand hinges, and controlled stance work.
- Progress one variable after 3–5 stable days and a good 24-hour response.
- If symptoms spike, regress range and remove the biggest irritant exercise temporarily.

Phase 2 is where your hip learns to trust itself again, one controlled step at a time.

Chapter 13: Strength Phase 3: Load and Power

What this chapter will change for you

You'll learn how to add real strength load without re-triggering hip irritation.

You'll build "usable power" (stand up fast, climb stairs confidently, return to running/lifting) without chasing intensity.

You'll get a Phase 3 menu with clear options for **glutes, adductors, hinge, squat, and lateral control**.

You'll know exactly how to progress load, speed, and volume, one lever at a time.

What "load and power" means in a hip-friendly context

Power doesn't mean plyometrics on day one. It means your hip can:

accept higher forces without flaring

- produce force smoothly (not with a protective jerk)
- transfer force through the pelvis without back/knee compensation
- tolerate faster movement when needed

In Phase 3, we keep the same philosophy: **calm, consistent, intelligently progressed.** We simply expand the range of "acceptable demand."

Phase 3 often applies to:

- returning to heavier lifting
- returning to running (especially speed/hills)
- sports that require changing direction
- people who want to feel athletic again, not just "less painful"

Phase 3 prerequisites (the "ready" signals)

You're ready for Phase 3 when most of these are true:

- Walking baseline is stable and you can add hills gradually without flare-ups
- Step-ups and step-downs are controlled without knee collapse or trunk lurch
- Split squats are comfortable through a moderate depth
- Kickstand hinge is strong and stable
- Single-leg stance is steady with minimal support
- Pain is low and predictable (not "spiky"), and returns to baseline within 24 hours

If you're not there, Phase 3 will feel like you're constantly managing symptoms. Phase 2 should feel boring before Phase 3 feels safe.

The Phase 3 principles (how we add intensity safely)

Think of "intensity" as three separate dials. You turn one at a time.

Load dial: more weight or band tension

Range dial: deeper positions (within tolerance)

Speed dial: faster intent (not sloppy speed)

Rule: Increase only one dial every 7–10 days, only if your 24-hour response is stable.

Also: power work is best done when you're fresh. If you're fatigued, you'll default to compensation.

The Phase 3 Menu (choose 5–7 per session)

Category A: Loaded squat pattern (hip-friendly depth)

1) Goblet squat to box (then gradually off box)

3–4 x 5–8 reps

Start with a box/chair that keeps you in a tolerable range.

Cues: "Sit between hips, ribs stacked, stand tall."
Regression: higher box, lighter load, slower tempo.
Progression: lower box, slightly heavier load, pause 1 second at the bottom (controlled).

Note: If deep flexion pinches, keep depth modest and build strength there. Depth returns later.

Category B: Loaded hinge (big strength payoff, usually hip-friendly)

2) Romanian deadlift (RDL) or hip hinge with weight

3–4 x 6–10 reps

Cues: "Hips back, spine quiet, feel hamstrings and glutes."
Regression: lighter load, shorter range (hands to thighs), slower tempo.
Progression: heavier load, longer range, or single-leg kickstand RDL with more load.

Hinge strength often reduces front-hip irritability by improving posterior support and load sharing.

Category C: Split squat / lunge strength (single-leg load)

3) Loaded split squat (goblet hold or suitcase hold)

3 x 6–8 each side

Cues: "Drop straight down, front heel heavy, pelvis level."
Regression: bodyweight, smaller range, more support.
Progression: add load, increase depth, or reduce support.

If knee symptoms appear, reduce range and focus on knee tracking; don't force "knee forward" depth.

Category D: Step strength (stairs translated into training)

4) Step-up with load (slow down, then add intent)

3 x 6–8 each side

Cues: "Quiet foot, drive through whole foot, stand tall at top."
Regression: lower step, lighter load, more support.

Progression: higher step or add a knee drive at top (only if control stays clean).

Category E: Lateral strength (hip + pelvis control under side load)

5) Lateral lunge to short range (supported if needed)

2–3 x 5–8 each side

Cues: "Step wide enough to feel inner thigh, hips back, push the floor away."
Regression: smaller step, use support, reduced depth.
Progression: wider step or add light load.

If groin is sensitive, keep this very small at first or stick with towel slides + split-stance adductor holds.

Category F: Hip abductors under load (outer hip durability)

6) Suitcase carry (anti-lean walking strength)

3–5 carries of 20–40 meters each side (or 20–40 seconds)

Hold a weight on one side and walk tall.

Cues: "Don't lean, ribs stacked, quiet steps."
Regression: lighter load, shorter carries.
Progression: heavier load or longer carries.

This is one of the most joint-friendly ways to build lateral hip and trunk control that transfers directly to walking/running.

Category G: Power entry points (low-risk, high value)

Power is about intent, not chaos. Start with "fast up, slow down" patterns.

7) Sit-to-stand with speed intent (controlled)

3 x 5–6 reps

Stand up with a quick, smooth effort; sit down slowly (3 seconds).

8) Step-up "pop" (only when stable)

2 x 5 each side

Push up with a bit more speed, still landing softly and controlled.

Rule: If speed makes you lose alignment, you're not ready for speed. Go back to slower reps.

Sample Phase 3 sessions (rotate)

Session A (Strength emphasis)

Goblet squat to box: 4 x 6

RDL: 4 x 8

Loaded split squat: 3 x 6/side

Suitcase carry: 4 x 30 sec/side

Optional calf raises: 2 x 12–15

Session B (Single-leg + lateral emphasis)

Step-up with load: 3 x 6–8/side

Kickstand RDL (heavier): 3 x 8/side

- Lateral lunge (short range): 2–3 x 6/side
- Towel slides or adductor holds: 2 sets
- Sit-to-stand speed intent: 3 x 5–6

Frequency: 2–4 days/week depending on goals and recovery.
If you're also returning to running, 2–3 strength days/week is usually plenty.

Progression rules (the "one dial" method)

Pick one dial to progress each week:

Week-to-week progression options

- Add **2–5% load** (or the smallest increment available)
- Add **1 rep per set** (up to your target range)
- Add **1 set** to one lift only
- Add **slightly more range** (a lower box, deeper split squat)

- Add **a little speed intent** to one exercise (not all)

When to hold

- Sleep is poor or stress is high
- You're sore beyond normal training soreness
- Walking or daily function feels more sensitive than usual

When to step down

- Sharp pain appears during lifts
- You develop a limp afterward
- Next day you're clearly worse (especially with night pain increase)

Step down by reducing range first, then volume, then load.

Common mistakes (and what to do instead)

Mistake: Adding load and speed together

Instead: choose one. Power comes from a stable base, not from rushing progression.

Mistake: Returning to deep ranges because "I should be able to"

Instead: earn depth. Deep hip flexion under load is a high-demand position. It's optional until it's tolerated.

Mistake: Skipping carries and lateral work

Instead: carries are a secret weapon for hip pain, low joint stress, high transfer.

Mistake: Training hard through "protective form"

If your trunk leans, knee caves, or you brace aggressively to survive reps, you're practicing compensation.
Instead: reduce load and rebuild clean reps. Quality is capacity.

Quick checklist / Action plan

- Confirm Phase 3 readiness: stable walking, controlled single-leg patterns, predictable symptoms.
- Train 2–4 days/week with a mix of squat, hinge, split squat, step, lateral work, and carries.
- Progress one dial at a time (load OR range OR speed) every 7–10 days if stable.
- Use power entry points: “fast up, slow down” before any jumping.
- If symptoms spike, step back range first, then volume, then load.

Phase 3 isn’t about proving anything. It’s about restoring the hip’s ability to handle real life, and real training, without fear.

Chapter 14: Squatting and Lunging Safely

What this chapter will change for you

- You'll learn how to adjust squats and lunges so they build capacity instead of provoking hip flare-ups.
- You'll know the difference between "**acceptable effort discomfort**" and "**stop-sign pain**" in deep hip positions.
- You'll get a clear technique system: **range → stance → trunk stack → knee track → tempo**.
- You'll have practical squat/lunge variations for desk workers, walkers, runners, and lifters, plus regressions.

Why squats and lunges trigger hip pain (and why they're still worth training)

Squats and lunges ask for a lot: hip flexion, rotation control, pelvic stability, and load tolerance. If your hip is flexion-sensitive, rotation-limited, or control-limited, deep loaded reps can feel "pinchy," unstable, or irritating.

That doesn't mean squats and lunges are bad for you. It means you need to adjust the variables so your hip can **earn** them.

The goal is not a textbook movement. The goal is a hip that can accept load through useful ranges without compensation or flare-ups.

The safety filter: what pain patterns mean "adjust now"

Use this during any squat/lunge work:

Green-light sensations (usually acceptable):

- mild muscular effort in glutes/quads/adductors
- mild stretch in hips that eases as you warm up
- 0–3/10 discomfort that doesn't linger into the next day

Yellow-light sensations (scale the set):

- pinching that appears at a specific depth
- discomfort that climbs rep to rep

form changes: knee diving, trunk lurching, foot gripping
Action: reduce depth, slow tempo, use support, or switch variation.

Red-light sensations (stop and reassess):

sharp pain, catching, giving way

pain that forces a limp

pain that spikes >5/10

next-day worsening that lasts beyond 24 hours
Action: stop the provoking version and regress for 1–2 weeks.

The technique system: adjust in this order

When a squat or lunge doesn't feel good, don't throw it out immediately. Change the variables in a sensible sequence:

Range (depth)

- **Stance** (width + toe angle)
- **Trunk stack** (ribs over pelvis)
- **Knee track** (over mid-foot)
- **Tempo** (slow down)
- **Load** (last)

Most people try to fix things by adding cues and forcing form. Usually the fix is simpler: change range and stance first.

Squatting Safely

Step 1: Pick the right squat "category" for your hip

Not everyone should start with a deep, free squat.

Category A: Chair/box squat (best starting point)

- Controls depth

- Reduces pinch risk
- Builds confidence fast

Category B: Counterbalance squat (helps rotation/stiffness)

- Holding a weight out front can improve trunk stacking and depth tolerance
- Works well for many people with stiffness

Category C: Free squat (earned later)

- Great, but not required early
- Add only when depth and control are stable

Squat setup: the 5-point checklist

Use this every time.

1. **Feet:** shoulder-width-ish, slight natural turnout (not forced straight)

Tripod foot: heel, base of big toe, base of little toe, steady, not gripping

Ribs stacked: exhale softly, keep ribcage from flaring

Sit between hips: think "down and back," not "collapse forward"

Knees track: over mid-foot (not rigid, not caving)

The "pinch problem": what to do if deep flexion irritates you

Front/groin pinching is often depth-related. Here's the conservative approach:

1) Reduce depth and train there for 2–4 weeks

Choose a box height that avoids pinch. Strength there often increases your depth later.

2) Adjust stance width slightly wider

Many hips tolerate flexion better with a slightly wider stance.

3) Increase toe turnout slightly (10–20%)

This can reduce internal rotation demand in deep flexion. Don't overdo it, excess turnout can stress the knee.

4) Use a counterbalance

Holding a light weight out front (goblet or plate) can help you stay stacked and reduce pinch.

5) Slow the tempo

3 seconds down, 1 second pause, smooth up. Tempo improves control and reduces "drop into the pinch."

If pinching persists even at modest depth, focus on hinge + split stance work for a few weeks and revisit later.

Squat variations (with regressions and progressions)

1) Sit-to-stand / box squat

- 3 x 6–10 reps
  - **Regression:** higher box, hands assistance
  - **Progression:** lower box, add load, slower

tempo

2) Goblet squat to box

3–4 x 5–8 reps

Regression: lighter load, higher box

Progression: lower box, brief pause, heavier load

3) Counterbalance squat (holding weight out)

2–3 x 6–8 reps

Good for: stiff hips, trunk control issues

Progression: remove counterbalance gradually

4) Hinge-biased "squat" (hybrid)

If squats irritate but you still want a leg pattern:

use a slightly higher hip position

hinge more

This keeps training going without provoking depth.

Lunging Safely

Why lunges are tricky (and powerful)

Lunges add:

- single-leg demand
- hip extension on the rear leg
- deeper hip flexion on the front leg
- balance and pelvic control

If your hip flexors are irritated or your pelvis control is limited, lunges can flare symptoms quickly. That's why we scale them.

Lunge setup: your stability anchors

- Use a wall/counter for support at first.
- Keep a "railroad track" stance, not a tightrope.

Keep your pelvis facing forward (avoid twisting).

Control the descent; don't drop fast.

Lunge progression ladder (safe order)

Level 1: Split-stance holds (Phase 1/2 bridge)

3 x 20–30 sec each side
Build position and tolerance first.

Level 2: Mini split squat (small bend and rise)

2–3 x 6–10 each side
Cue: "Down a little, up a little, quiet pelvis."

Level 3: Full split squat (moderate depth)

3 x 6–8 each side
Add depth only if no pinching or next-day flare.

Level 4: Reverse lunge (often the most hip-friendly dynamic lunge)

Stepping back tends to be easier on the knee and often more controllable than stepping forward.

2–3 x 5–8 each side

Level 5: Forward lunge / walking lunge (highest demand)

Great later, but not necessary early. Add only when you own Levels 1–4.

Common lunge issues (and fixes)

Issue 1: Front-hip pinch on the working leg

Fix: reduce depth, slightly widen stance, use reverse lunge or split squat to a target, keep ribs stacked.

Issue 2: Rear-leg hip flexor pain

Fix: shorten stance, reduce depth, keep pelvis gently tucked (5–10%), add more glute support work (Ch.7), avoid aggressive hip flexor stretching.

Issue 3: Knee pain or knee dive

Fix: “railroad track” stance, slow tempo, reduce range, strengthen lateral hip and adductors (Ch.7–9).

Issue 4: Balance limitation

Fix: use support. Balance demand is optional; hip loading is the point.

Technique is not rigid, it’s repeatable

A calm reminder: different hips like different stances. Some people squat better wider; some better narrower. Some need a little toe turnout. The goal isn’t to match a template. The goal is to find the version that:

- stays within tolerance
- improves capacity over weeks
- reduces compensation in back and knees

That’s “safe technique.”

Common mistakes (and smarter alternatives)

Mistake: Forcing deep squats because "I should be able to"

Instead: train pain-free depth now. Depth is earned by strength and tolerance.

Mistake: Treating every pinch as damage

Instead: treat it as a signal to adjust range/stance/tempo and build capacity.

Mistake: Doing high-rep lunges when control is shaky

Instead: fewer reps, slower tempo, more support.

Mistake: Holding your breath and bracing hard

Instead: breathe steadily. Excess bracing often increases hip guarding.

Quick checklist / Action plan

- Use the adjustment order: **range → stance → stack → knee track → tempo → load**.
- Start squats with a box/chair; start lunges with split-stance holds.
- If pinching appears, reduce depth and use a slightly wider stance + gentle toe turnout.
- Prefer reverse lunges and split squats before forward/walking lunges.
- Progress one variable at a time, using the 24-hour check.

Squats and lunges don't need to be feared or worshipped. They're tools. Your job is to choose the version that your hip can tolerate today, and that it can grow from tomorrow.

Chapter 15: Running Mechanics and Hip Load

What this chapter will change for you

You'll understand why running can flare hip pain even when walking feels fine, and how to reduce the "magnifier effect."

You'll learn the few running variables that matter most for hip load: **stride, cadence, trunk position, and terrain**.

You'll get a practical return-to-run framework using **baseline + tolerance + 24-hour check**.

You'll know what to adjust first when pain appears, without chasing perfect form.

Why running is a magnifier (not a moral test)

Running isn't "bad for hips." It's just high-frequency single-leg loading. Each step is a landing, a brief single-leg stance, and a push-off, repeated hundreds or thousands of times.

If your hip currently has:

reduced **single-leg control**,

limited **hip extension** tolerance,

irritated lateral tissues, or

a capacity gap in adductors/glutes,

...running amplifies it quickly. The good news is that this also means running improves when you reduce peak load and rebuild capacity, calmly and systematically.

The three dials of running load (turn one at a time)

Think like a coach, not a gambler. Running load has three main dials:

Dial 1: Volume (how much)

Minutes per run, runs per week, and total weekly time.

Dial 2: Intensity (how hard)

Speed, hills, intervals, surges, and "running on tired legs."

Dial 3: Mechanics (how you distribute load)

Stride length, cadence, trunk/pelvis control, and foot placement.

Rule: When returning from hip pain, change only one dial at a time. If you increase volume, keep intensity and terrain easy. If you add hills, keep volume stable.

Before you run: "Are you ready today?" (a 60-second readiness check)

Running readiness is not about being fearless. It's about predictable tolerance.

You're more likely ready to try a run if:

- You can walk briskly for **20–30 minutes** without limping and without next-day worsening
- You can do **step-ups** and **split squats** (moderate depth) with steady knee tracking
- Single-leg stance feels steady for **30 seconds** with minimal wobble
- Your hip symptoms are **stable** (not spiking day to day)

If you're missing multiple items, your hip may benefit from more Phase 2/3 work before you reintroduce running volume.

A simple running form audit (keep it human)

You don't need a lab. You need awareness of a few patterns that commonly increase hip irritation.

During an easy jog, notice:

1) Stride: are you reaching?

Overstriding (foot landing far in front of you) often increases front-hip irritation and joint load.

Better target: slightly shorter stride.

2) Cadence: are steps slow and "bounding"?

A low cadence often increases time and load per step.

Better target: slightly quicker steps without speeding up.

3) Trunk: are you leaning a lot or swaying?

A big side-to-side sway can increase lateral hip demand. A big forward bend can increase hip flexor workload.

Better target: a "quiet trunk," with gentle forward lean from the ankles (not a fold at the waist).

4) Foot turnout: are you running duck-footed?

A lot of turnout can be a protection strategy that reduces hip rotation demand, but it can also shift load to knee/outer hip.

Better target: reduce turnout by 10–20% (don't force straight).

The cue menu (choose ONE cue at a time)

Use cues like seasoning, not a full recipe. Pick one and test it for 30–60 seconds.

Cue A: "Shorter, quicker steps"

This reduces peak hip load and overstride without you thinking about posture.

Cue B: "Run quietly"

Softer foot contact often correlates with better control and less bracing.

Cue C: "Head stays level"

A simple way to reduce trunk sway. Imagine a smooth forward glide.

Cue D: "Push the ground behind you"

Helpful if you feel front-hip gripping. It encourages posterior chain contribution without forcing extension.

Cue E: "Railroad tracks"

If you feel twisting or knee dive, imagine your feet landing on parallel tracks instead of crossing over midline.

If a cue increases tension or makes you feel robotic, drop it. The goal is a slightly better pattern, not a new personality.

Hills, speed, and cambered roads: load multipliers

A flat easy run is one thing. Add hills and you've changed the entire demand profile.

Hills

Uphills increase hip flexor and glute demand.

Downhills increase landing forces and control demands.

Rule: return to hills last. Start flat.

Speedwork

Strides, intervals, and tempo runs increase peak forces and often expose capacity gaps.

Rule: rebuild easy volume first, then add speed later, and only if your hip is stable for weeks.

Cambered roads (slanted surfaces)

These can overload lateral hip tissues, especially if one leg is always "downhill."

Rule: avoid long cambered runs early. Choose flat paths or switch sides.

The return-to-run system: baseline → build → consolidate

This is the conservative model that protects you from the classic cycle: feel good → do too much → flare → rest → repeat.

Step 1: Set your run baseline

Your baseline run is the smallest run dose you can repeat that:

- stays within **0–3/10** discomfort
- doesn't change your gait (no limping)
- returns you near baseline within **24 hours**

For many people, that baseline is run/walk.

Example baselines (choose the easiest that fits):

- 10–15 minutes total: 1 min jog / 1 min walk x 5–7 rounds
- 15–20 minutes total: 2 min jog / 1 min walk x 5 rounds
- 10 minutes continuous jog (only if symptoms are low and stable)

If you're unsure, start with 1:1 run/walk. It's not "less real." It's controlled dosing.

Step 2: Build one variable at a time

After **3–5 stable days** (and a stable 24-hour response), progress one variable:

Add 1–2 minutes total time, OR

Add one extra interval round, OR

Increase jog interval slightly (e.g., 1 min → 90 sec) while keeping total time similar

Do not progress volume and intensity in the same week.

Step 3: Consolidate

Every 3rd or 4th week, keep volume steady (or even slightly lower) to let tissues adapt. Consistency beats constant escalation.

The 24-hour rule for runners (your guardrail)

Use this after every run session:

Green response: mild soreness that resolves and you feel normal next day → continue.

Yellow response: noticeable soreness or stiffness next day, but no limp and it settles within 24 hours → repeat the same dose (don't progress).

Red response: limp, sharp pain, night pain increase, or clear next-day worsening lasting >24 hours → regress.

Regression options (choose one):

- Reduce total time by 20–30%
- Return to run/walk if you tried continuous
- Remove hills/speed entirely
- Add an extra rest day between runs and keep strength work steady

A flare-up is feedback about dose, not proof you're damaged.

Where strength fits while you return to running

Your running improves fastest when strength supports it, not competes with it.

A simple pairing:

- Run 2–3 days/week (easy)
- Strength 2–3 days/week (Phase 2 or Phase 3 depending on readiness)
- Avoid heavy leg strength the day before your longest run early on

If your hip gets reactive, keep strength but reduce running dose first. Strength builds capacity; running tests it.

Troubleshooting by symptom location (practical patterns)

Front hip / groin irritation during or after runs

Common drivers: overstride, hills too soon, deep flexion sensitivity, hip flexor/adductor overload.
Try: shorter stride + slightly quicker steps, flatter routes, keep runs shorter, maintain glute/adductor work.

Lateral hip ache (outer hip) during longer runs

Common drivers: pelvic drop, trunk sway, cambered roads, weak lateral hip endurance.
Try: reduce distance, add suitcase carries and wall press holds, run on flatter surfaces, avoid slanted roads.

Hip + back tightness after running

Common drivers: extension borrowed from low back, insufficient glute contribution, excessive arching.
Try: "ribs stacked" before runs, hinge and bridge work, shorter stride, avoid sprinting/hills early.

Common mistakes (and what to do instead)

Mistake: Using a "good day" to justify a big run

Do instead: treat good days as proof your baseline is working, then progress gradually.

Mistake: Fixing form by forcing everything at once

Do instead: one cue, one change, short test.

Mistake: Returning to speed because you miss it

Do instead: earn speed by building easy volume + Phase 3 strength first. Speed is the last dial.

Mistake: Running through a limp

Do instead: stop the run, walk home, and regress next session. Limping is a clear sign the dose is too high today.

Quick checklist / Action plan

- Establish a run baseline (often run/walk) that respects tolerance and the 24-hour check.
- Keep early runs flat and easy; treat hills and speed as multipliers.
- Use one cue at a time: **shorter/quicker**, **run quietly**, **head level**, **push behind**, **railroad tracks**.
- Pair running with Phase 2/3 strength to build capacity, not just test it.
- If symptoms spike: reduce volume first, remove hills/speed, and return to run/walk.

You don't need perfect mechanics to run again. You need a repeatable dose, steadier single-leg control, and patient progression. That's how hips rebuild trust.

Chapter 16: Hip Pain and Back Pain Connection

What this chapter will change for you

You'll understand the most common ways hip limitations shift load into the low back, without blaming your posture.

You'll learn how to tell if your back is "**helping**" because the hip is missing options, versus a back-driven problem.

You'll get a practical plan to reduce back strain by improving hip contribution: **stack → hinge → rotate → walk**.

You'll have simple decision rules for training when both areas are sensitive.

The big picture: the back often compensates for the hip

The hip and low back are teammates. They share the job of moving you through space, especially during bending, walking, stairs, running, and lifting.

When hip motion or hip strength is limited, the back often steps in. That doesn't mean your back is "weak." It means your system is trying to keep you moving with the options it has.

Hip-to-back compensation usually shows up in three ways:

- the back moves more because the hip moves less
- the back stiffens to create stability the hip isn't providing
- the back absorbs rotation and extension because the hip can't

The goal isn't to "protect the back by never moving it." The goal is to **restore sharing**: hip takes its portion of the job again.

The three common hip-to-back pathways

Pathway 1: Extension deficit → back over-arches

If hip extension is limited (often from prolonged sitting, hip flexor irritation, or protective guarding), you may get extension by arching the low back, especially during:

- walking fast or uphill
- running
- standing up from a chair
- lunges (rear leg extension demand)

Clues:

- back feels tight after walking or standing
- you feel "compression" in low back during lunges
- your front hip feels grippy and your back arches to get stride

Plan: restore small amounts of hip extension tolerance and strengthen glutes so the back doesn't have to create the motion.

Pathway 2: Rotation deficit → back twists instead

If hip rotation is limited (especially internal rotation), the pelvis still needs to rotate during walking. If the hip can't contribute, the spine often rotates more.

Clues:

- back tightness with turning, rolling in bed, long walks
- one-sided low back soreness that correlates with hip stiffness
- knee irritation shows up too (because rotation gets borrowed down the chain)

Plan: gentle hip rotation mobility (Chapter 6) + single-leg control (Chapter 12) to reduce "borrowed twist."

Pathway 3: Control deficit → back braces to stabilize

When the hip doesn't feel stable under load, especially on one leg, the trunk often braces harder. This can create a persistent back tension pattern.

Clues:

- you feel you must “hold your breath” to move
- back gets tired during stairs or carries
- lateral hip pain and back tightness appear together after longer days

Plan: build pelvic stability (Ch.7–9) and use carries/hinges to train stability without over-bracing.

Is it hip-driven, back-driven, or shared? (a practical screen)

This is not a medical diagnosis. It’s a helpful sorting tool.

संकेत it’s more hip-driven (back is compensating)

- Back discomfort increases after hip-loading tasks (stairs, hills, long walks)
- Hip mobility tests are clearly limited or sensitive (Chapter 6)
- Gentle hip-focused work improves back comfort

Back pain feels more like fatigue/tightness than sharp nerve symptoms

संकेत it may be more back-driven

Back pain is the primary limiter even when hips feel okay

Symptoms radiate down the leg with numbness/tingling or progressive weakness

Coughing/sneezing strongly affects pain

You have red flags (Chapter 3)

Most common reality: shared

Hip and back influence each other. We still start with conservative steps that improve load sharing, because they tend to help both.

The practical system: Stack → Hinge → Rotate → Walk

This is the sequence that often reduces both hip and back irritation.

1) Stack (ribs over pelvis)

When your ribcage flares up and pelvis tips forward, hip extension gets harder and the back takes more load.

Stack reset (90 seconds):

4 slow breaths (long exhales)

gentle pelvic tuck 5–10%

stand up and keep the same “stack” feeling

Use this before walks, lifts, or long sitting transitions.

---

2) Hinge (move at hips, not through the spine)

Hinging trains the hip to do what it’s designed to do: accept load while the spine stays calm.

Hip hinge to wall

2–3 x 8–12 slow reps
Cue: “Hips back, ribs quiet, shins mostly

vertical."

Loaded hinge (Phase 3)

RDLs or good morning pattern with light load
Rule: if you feel it mainly in the low back, reduce range and load; make the movement smaller and cleaner.

Hinge strength often reduces back "helping" more than any stretch does.

---

3) Rotate (give rotation back to the hip)

Rotation doesn't have to be aggressive. It has to be **available**.

Gentle seated hip rotations

2 x 6 each direction per side
Stay far from pinching.

90/90 supported switches

2 x 6 per side
Support with hands; keep it calm.

Your goal is to reintroduce rotation options so walking and turning don't steal from the spine.

---

4) Walk (practice the sharing in real life)

Walking is where hip-back sharing is tested.

If your back tightens during walking:

- shorten stride slightly
- use "push the ground behind you"
- keep ribs stacked
- reduce hills early
- keep walking dose at baseline until next-day response is stable

A steady baseline walk often helps back pain when the hip is the driver, because it trains rhythm and load sharing.

The “two-zone” approach when both hip and back are sensitive

If you’re in a flare where both areas are reactive, your training needs simpler boundaries.

Zone 1: Calm exposure (daily, short)

- 5–10 minutes total
- mobility + breathing + easy hinges
- aim for “less guarded,” not “more flexible”

Example Zone 1 set:

- 4 breaths (stack)
- hip hinge to wall x 8
- gentle 90/90 rotations x 6/side
- 5-minute easy walk

Zone 2: Strength (2–3 days/week)

Choose exercises that load hips without forcing spine extension/rotation.

Good options:

- sit-to-stand / box squat
- split-stance holds or shallow split squats
- bridge holds
- suitcase carries (if tolerated)
- RDLs with light load and short range

Avoid early on (if reactive):

- deep flexion with heavy load
- high-rep twisting/lunging patterns
- sprinting/hills

Common mistakes (and what to do instead)

Mistake: Treating the back like glass

Instead: keep the back calm, not immobile. Build hip contribution so the back doesn't have to overwork.

Mistake: Stretching the back aggressively when the hip is the limiter

Instead: hinge and hip mobility often reduce back tightness more effectively than back stretching alone.

Mistake: Over-bracing all day

Instead: learn "just enough" brace during tasks, and let the system breathe again between efforts. Constant bracing increases guarding.

Mistake: Forcing long strides to "open the hip"

Instead: earn extension gradually. Overstriding often increases both front hip irritation and back arching.

Quick checklist / Action plan

If back pain is present, assume the hip-back relationship matters and train load sharing.

- Use the sequence: **stack → hinge → rotate → walk** (most days).
- Train strength 2–3 days/week with hip-friendly patterns (box squat, split stance, hinge, carries).
- Use walking cues: shorter stride, push behind, ribs stacked.
- Seek evaluation if you have red flags or progressive neurological symptoms.

When hips do their share, backs often calm down, not because you "protected" the back, but because you restored teamwork.

Chapter 17: Hip Pain and Knee Pain Connection

What this chapter will change for you

You'll understand how hip capacity (or the lack of it) changes knee load during walking, stairs, squats, and running.

You'll learn the two most common knee-compensation patterns: **knee collapse** and **knee overwork from stiffness**.

You'll get a practical "hip-to-knee protection" plan:

foot → knee track → pelvis control → task dosing.

You'll know when knee pain is likely a **dose problem** versus a sign you should seek evaluation.

The knee is a hardworking middle joint

The knee is designed to hinge and manage forces, especially in forward/backward motion. But it's not designed to be the primary controller of pelvic position or hip rotation. When the hip isn't sharing load, the knee often becomes the "middle manager" for problems above and below.

That's why knee pain can show up alongside hip pain, even when the knee itself didn't "do anything wrong."

The goal of this chapter is not to diagnose your knee. It's to reduce unnecessary knee stress by improving how the chain shares load.

The two main pathways: how hips overload knees

Pathway 1: Hip control deficit → knee collapse and overuse

When the lateral hip muscles (glute med/deep stabilizers) fatigue or don't coordinate well, the thigh can drift inward during single-leg tasks. The knee follows.

This shows up as:

- knee diving inward on stairs, step-downs, lunges
- medial knee ache or patellofemoral discomfort (front of knee)

- lateral hip ache plus knee irritation after longer walks/runs
- foot arch collapsing or foot gripping to “save the knee”

Translation: the knee is trying to stabilize what the hip should stabilize.

Pathway 2: Hip stiffness/rotation limits → knee twists instead

If hip rotation is limited, especially internal rotation, the body still needs rotation during gait and squats. If the hip can’t provide it, rotation often shows up at the knee or foot.

This can feel like:

- knee discomfort during turning, pivoting, or downhill walking
- “tight” IT band sensation (often really lateral hip/thigh tension)
- knee ache during squats at certain depths

- the foot turning out more to avoid hip rotation demand

Translation: the knee gets asked to rotate more than it wants to.

A simple chain check: what do you see when you step down?

Use a low step. Hold a counter lightly.

Step-down snapshot (5 reps each side):

- Stand on a step and tap the other heel to the floor slowly.
  Watch:

- does the knee drift inward?
- does the pelvis drop or hike?
- does the trunk lean a lot?
- does the foot collapse/grip?

If knee dives inward: hip abductor/adductor balance and pelvis control are likely key.
If foot collapses first: foot/calf strength and foot control may be part of the solution.
If trunk leans dramatically: you may be unloading hip abductors; reduce range and build stability.

This is not a "form test." It's information.

The practical system: Foot → Knee track → Pelvis control → Task dosing

When knee and hip both complain, we simplify the priorities.

1) Foot: give the knee a stable base

You don't need perfect arches. You need a foot that can accept load without collapsing into panic.

Foot "tripod" cue (during standing tasks):

heel

base of big toe

base of little toe

Keep these three points heavy and steady.

Supported calf raises: 2–3 x 10–15
Strong calves reduce knee load during walking and running by improving shock absorption and push-off mechanics.

Note: If foot work aggravates symptoms, reduce volume and keep it gentle.

---

2) Knee tracking: "steady, not stiff"

A knee that collapses inward increases stress. A knee forced rigidly outward can also feel bad. We want a steady midline path.

Tracking cue: "Knee over mid-foot."
Not perfect. Just consistent.

Best early drill: sit-to-stand

3 x 6–10

Focus on even pressure through feet and steady knee path.

Best Phase 2 drill: step-up with slow lower

2–3 x 6–8 each side
Slow lowering builds control and tolerance.

---

3) Pelvis control: the hip's biggest gift to the knee

This is where Chapter 7–9 work pays off.

Lateral wall press holds: 2–3 x 15–25 sec/side
Builds lateral hip endurance without knee strain.

Supported single-leg stance: 3 x 20–40 sec/side
Pelvis "level enough," knee soft.

Adductor support (pillow squeezes or towel slides):
Inner thigh strength helps prevent pelvic drift and knee collapse during loaded flexion.

---

4) Task dosing: reduce knee irritation by respecting volume

Many knee flare-ups are dose problems, not structural disasters.

Dose multipliers for knees:

- downhill walking and running
- deep squats/lunges under fatigue
- high step volume (stairs, hiking)
- sudden increases in walking or running time

Rule: if knee symptoms increase, adjust **volume** and **depth** before changing everything else.

Knee-friendly modifications for common tasks

Stairs

If stairs hurt:

- use a handrail temporarily (not forever, just as a bridge)
- take slower steps and keep foot pressure steady
- avoid rushing down stairs early on (descending is higher control demand)

Train: step-ups with slow lowering 2–3 days/week.

Squats

If squats cause knee pain:

- use a box/chair to limit depth
- widen stance slightly if comfortable
- reduce load and slow tempo (3 seconds down)

Remember: depth is a variable. Train in your tolerated depth.

Lunges

If lunges irritate the knee:

- start with split-stance holds
- use reverse lunges instead of forward lunges
- keep shin angle more vertical at first
- reduce range and use support

Running

If knee pain appears during return-to-run:

- shorten stride slightly and increase cadence a bit
- keep runs flat and easy
- reduce weekly volume and build strength support

When knee pain needs medical care (quick safety notes)

Seek evaluation sooner if you have:

- significant swelling, heat, or redness around the knee
- inability to bear weight or the knee gives way repeatedly
- locking (true inability to straighten/bend)
- a traumatic injury with immediate swelling
- fever/systemic symptoms
- rapidly worsening pain despite conservative dosing

If knee pain is persistent and unclear, getting assessed is smart. The goal is clarity, not toughing it out.

Common mistakes (and what to do instead)

Mistake: Trying to "fix the knee" without training the hip

Instead: treat the knee as part of the chain. Hip control often reduces knee symptoms more than knee isolation work alone.

Mistake: Forcing knees outward aggressively

Instead: aim for steady tracking over mid-foot. Too much forced outward cueing can create new irritation.

Mistake: Ignoring calves and feet

Instead: add basic calf raises and foot tripod awareness. Small inputs, big payoff.

Mistake: Increasing walking/running volume while knee is already irritated

Instead: reduce dose first, then rebuild with strength and gradual progression.

Quick checklist / Action plan

- Check your step-down: knee dive, pelvis drop, foot collapse, note what shows up first.
- Strengthen the base: calf raises + tripod foot in standing tasks.
- Train knee tracking with box squats and step-ups (slow lowering).
- Build pelvis control with wall press holds, single-leg stance, and adductor work.
- Dose tasks conservatively: reduce downhill, deep fatigue reps, and sudden volume spikes.

When hips regain control, knees often stop acting like the emergency stabilizer. Your job is to rebuild the chain so load is shared, quietly, consistently, and with patience.

Chapter 18: Managing Flare-Ups

What this chapter will change for you

- You'll stop treating flare-ups as failure and start treating them as **dose feedback**.
- You'll learn a simple flare-up playbook: **settle → protect → maintain → rebuild**.
- You'll get clear step-down rules for walking, strength, and mobility, and clear "return rules."
- You'll know when a flare-up is *not* a typical flare-up and should be evaluated.

What a flare-up is (and what it isn't)

A flare-up is a temporary increase in pain, stiffness, or sensitivity that reduces function, often after a spike in load, a long sitting day, a new exercise, poor sleep, or stress.

A flare-up is usually:

- a sign your **current dose** exceeded tolerance

- a combination of tissue sensitivity + protective nervous system response
- reversible with calm, consistent management

A flare-up is not automatically:

- new damage
- proof that movement is unsafe
- a reason to start over from zero

Your goal is to respond quickly and calmly so the flare is shorter and less disruptive.

The two types of flare-ups (so you choose the right response)

Type 1: “I did too much” flare (dose flare)

Common triggers:

- longer walk than baseline

hills/stairs volume spike

deeper squats/lunges than usual

adding load and speed together

long sitting then sudden activity

Pattern: symptoms increase after the event and linger 24–72 hours.

Best response: step down dose, keep movement present, rebuild.

Type 2: "Life hit me" flare (recovery flare)

Common triggers:

poor sleep

high stress

illness

travel / long sitting

sudden schedule change

Pattern: symptoms feel more diffuse, tolerance is lower across many activities.

Best response: reduce total training demand, prioritize calming routines, then return gradually.

Both types are real. Both respond to structure.

First: the flare-up safety check

Before you assume it's a typical flare, quickly screen for "not normal for you."

Seek medical evaluation if you have:

- inability to bear weight or a new significant limp you can't reduce
- major trauma (fall/collision)
- fever, redness/warmth, feeling unwell
- rapidly worsening pain, severe night pain that escalates
- new neurological symptoms (numbness, progressive weakness, bowel/bladder changes)

significant swelling or bruising

If none of those are present, proceed with the flare-up playbook.

The Flare-Up Playbook: Settle → Protect → Maintain → Rebuild

Step 1: Settle (0–24 hours)

Your first job is to reduce threat. Not by freezing, by lowering intensity and giving the system predictable input.

Settle routine (6–10 minutes, 1–2x/day)

Breathing stack reset (2 minutes)

slow exhale, ribs soften down, gentle pelvic stacking

Gentle weight shifts (60 seconds)

side-to-side, small range

Short walk or march (2–5 minutes)

flat, easy, stop if limp increases

Isometric support (choose 1)

Bridge hold: 3 x 15–20 sec

Pillow squeeze: 4 x 15–20 sec

Wall press hold: 2–3 x 15 sec/side

Rules:

keep discomfort 0–3/10 and non-sharp

stop if gait worsens

the goal is "settled," not "stretched"

Helpful mindset: treat it like turning down the volume, not deleting the song.

Step 2: Protect (24–72 hours) - step-down rules

Now you adjust your training and daily load so the flare doesn't snowball.

Step-down rule for walking

Pick the option that matches your flare severity:

- **Mild flare:** reduce walking time by **20–30%**; keep flat; keep pace easy.
- **Moderate flare:** reduce by **40–60%** OR split into 2–3 short walks.
- **High irritability flare:** do only short "movement snacks" (1–3 minutes) every few hours if tolerated.

Non-negotiable: don't practice a limp. If you limp, your walk dose is too high today.

Step-down rule for strength training

Keep strength present, but change the dose.

- Remove the most provocative exercises first (often: step-downs, deep lunges, lateral lunges, heavy squats, hills/sprints).
- Shift toward **isometrics + short range** for 3–7 days.

A safe flare-up strength menu (2–3 days/week):

- Sit-to-stand to a higher chair: 2 x 6–8 (slow)
- Split-stance hold with support: 2 x 20 sec/side
- Bridge hold: 3 x 15–25 sec
- Wall press hold: 2 x 15–25 sec/side
- Pillow squeeze: 4 x 15–20 sec

If any drill spikes pain sharply or worsens next day, reduce range/effort.

Step-down rule for mobility

When irritated, “more mobility” can be too much.

- Keep mobility to **gentle, short-range** drills (5–8 minutes/day).

- Avoid long end-range holds and aggressive stretching.
- Favor rocking motions and supported rotations.

Step 3: Maintain (days 3–7) - keep the floor from dropping out

This step is about staying connected to your routine so you don't lose confidence.

The minimum effective dose template (10–15 minutes/day)

- 2 minutes breathing stack
- 3–5 minutes easy walk (or 2 x 2–3 minute walks)
- 6–8 minutes of 2–3 supportive drills (isometrics + one mobility)

Your goal: symptoms trend toward baseline again, even if slowly.

Progress marker: you can move through the day with less guarding and less unpredictability.

Step 4: Rebuild (return rules)

Return rules prevent the classic mistake: you feel better and jump straight back to peak volume.

Return rule 1: Two stable days first

Before you progress, you want **two consecutive days** where:

- you walk without limping
- daily pain is near baseline
- sleep isn't clearly worsened by symptoms

Return rule 2: Reintroduce one stressor at a time

Choose one:

- increase walk time slightly
- add back one strength exercise
- increase range slightly

add a small load

Do not reintroduce hills/speed and deep strength progressions in the same week.

Return rule 3: Use the "half-step" progression

After a flare, your first progression should be **half** of what you'd normally add.

Example:

- If you usually add 5 minutes to a walk, add 2–3 minutes instead.
- If you usually add a set, add 1–2 reps instead.
- If you usually lower the squat box height, lower it one notch and keep load the same.

Return rule 4: The 24-hour check still governs everything

If next day worsens, step back immediately, don't wait for it to "prove" itself.

Why flare-ups often cluster (and how to stop the pattern)

If you're flaring every 1–2 weeks, it's usually one of these:

Your baseline is too high
You're living above tolerance and paying for it regularly.

You're progressing too many variables at once
Volume + hills + new strength work is a common combo.

You're not accounting for recovery capacity
Bad sleep and stress reduce tolerance. The same workout becomes a different dose.

You're chasing stretches instead of building strength
If stretching is your main tool, you may not be building the capacity that prevents flares.

Fix: lower baseline slightly, progress one dial at a time, keep strength consistent, and use step-down rules quickly.

Common mistakes (and what to do instead)

Mistake: Full rest until you feel perfect

Instead: keep movement present at a minimum effective dose. Capacity hates long gaps.

Mistake: "Testing" the hip repeatedly during a flare

Instead: choose one daily check (short walk) and stop poking the bear.

Mistake: Trying to stretch the flare away

Instead: settle with breath + isometrics + short-range mobility.

Mistake: Returning to peak training the moment it feels better

Instead: two stable days, then half-step progression.

Quick checklist / Action plan

- Screen red flags first (weight-bearing, trauma, systemic signs, neuro changes).
- Use the playbook: **Settle → Protect → Maintain → Rebuild**.
- Step down walking (20–60% depending on severity) and avoid limping.
- Shift strength to isometrics and short ranges for 3–7 days.
- Return with two stable days + one stressor at a time + half-step progressions.

Flare-ups are part of building capacity. The difference between people who get stuck and people who improve is not “never flaring.” It’s knowing exactly what to do when they do.

Chapter 19: 30-Day Hip Strength Plan

What this chapter will change for you

- You'll have a complete **30-day structure** that builds hip strength without guessing day to day.
- You'll know exactly how to set your **baseline**, then progress load safely using simple rules.
- You'll get three tracks (sensitive / steady / athletic) so the plan fits your current **tolerance**.
- You'll have built-in "if-this-then-that" adjustments for **flare-ups**, busy weeks, and return-to-running/lifting.

The point of a 30-day plan: consistency beats intensity

Thirty days is long enough to create real change, and short enough to stay focused. Your goal is not to crush workouts. Your goal is to repeat a dose your hip can adapt to.

You're building three things at the same time:

Capacity (the hip can handle more without irritation)

Single-leg control (walking, stairs, running feel steadier)

Confidence (you trust movement again)

This plan uses the phases you've already learned:

Phase 1: foundational stability (Chapter 11)

Phase 2: single-leg control (Chapter 12)

Phase 3: load and power (Chapter 13)

You'll progress through them in a conservative way, guided by your symptoms, not your ambition.

Step 1: Choose your starting track (don't overthink it)

Pick the track that matches your last 7–10 days.

Track A - Sensitive (irritable or recently flared)

walking baseline is low or inconsistent

stairs provoke symptoms

flare-ups happen easily
Plan: 3 strength days/week, low-to-moderate volume, more isometrics.

Track B - Steady (most people)

walking is stable without limping

you tolerate Phase 1 work well

symptoms are predictable and settle within 24 hours
Plan: 4 strength days/week (2 main + 2 lighter), gradual Phase 2 work.

Track C - Athletic (returning to running/lifting)

Phase 2 drills feel solid

you recover well

symptoms are low and stable
Plan: 4 strength days/week with a Phase 3 emphasis + careful speed/power entry points.

If you choose a track and it proves too much, that's not failure, just information. Step down one track for a week.

Step 2: Your non-negotiables (the guardrails)

- **Pain rule:** keep training discomfort **0–3/10**, non-sharp.
- **Gait rule:** no limping practice. If you limp, reduce dose.
- **24-hour rule:** you should return near baseline within **24 hours**.
- **One dial at a time:** change only one variable (range OR load OR volume OR speed) every 7–10 days.

The 30-Day Weekly Structure (Weeks 1–4)

Week 1: Stabilize and “earn the right”

Focus: Phase 1 patterns + calm walking baseline.
Strength days: 3–4 depending on track.
Goal: leave every session feeling better coordinated, not wrecked.

Strength Sessions (Week 1)

Session A (Phase 1 foundation)

Sit-to-stand / box squat: 3 x 6–10

Hinge to wall: 2–3 x 8–12

Supported split-stance hold: 3 x 20–30 sec/side

Bridge hold: 3 x 20–30 sec

Lateral wall press hold: 2–3 x 15–25 sec/side

Session B (Phase 1 + inner hip support)

Sit-to-stand (slower): 3 x 6–8

Pillow squeeze isometric: 4–6 x 20 sec

Side-lying abduction hold: 2 x 15–25 sec/side

Hinge to wall: 2 x 10

Calf raises: 2 x 12–15

Walking: baseline dose on flat terrain.

Week 2: Build control (introduce Phase 2 carefully)

Focus: supported single-leg work with modest volume.
Goal: stairs and longer walks feel steadier.

Strength Sessions (Week 2)

Session A (Phase 1 → 2 bridge)

Supported single-leg stance: 3 x 20–40 sec/side

Step-up + slow lower (low step): 2–3 x 6–8/side

Supported split squat (shallow): 2–3 x 6–10/side

Bridge reps or holds: 2–3 sets

Wall press hold OR band walk (light): 2 sets

Session B (Control + adductors)

Toe-touch single-leg stance: 3 x 30 sec/side

Towel slides: 2 x 6–10/side

Sit-to-stand: 3 x 6–10

Pillow squeeze: 4 x 20 sec

Calf raises: 2 x 12–15

Walking: baseline + small progress only if Week 1 was stable (10–20% max).

Week 3: Single-leg capacity week (Phase 2 emphasis)

Focus: more repeatable single-leg strength without increasing speed yet.
Goal: you feel "less wobbly" and recover faster.

Strength Sessions (Week 3)

Session A (Single-leg strength)

Step-up + slow lower: 3 x 6–8/side

Kickstand RDL: 3 x 6–10/side

Supported split squat (moderate depth if tolerated): 3 x 6–8/side

Lateral wall press OR band walk: 2 sets

Optional: bridge reps 2 x 10–12

Session B (Lateral control day - conservative)

Supported single-leg stance: 3 x 30–45 sec/side

Lateral step-down (small range): 2 x 5–8/side

Towel slides: 2 x 8/side

Side-lying abduction hold: 2 x 15–20 sec/side

Calf raises: 2 x 12–15

Walking: keep stable; don't add hills and volume in the same week.

Week 4: Consolidate + introduce Phase 3 elements (only if earned)

Focus: add load (or speed intent) *carefully* OR consolidate if you're still adapting.
Goal: stronger patterns with the same calm control.

Option 1: Consolidation week (recommended if you're uncertain)

Repeat Week 3 sessions with **no progressions**, aiming for cleaner reps and better recovery.

Option 2: Phase 3 "entry" (Track C, or stable Track B)

Choose **one** Phase 3 dial to introduce:

Dial: Load (preferred first)

Goblet squat to box: 3–4 x 5–8

RDL (light/moderate): 3–4 x 6–10
Keep single-leg work stable (don't progress everything).

Dial: Speed intent (only if symptoms are very stable)

Sit-to-stand "fast up, slow down": 3 x 5–6

Everything else stays the same.

Walking/running: if returning to running, keep runs easy and keep strength stable (don't add load and run volume together).

Your weekly schedule (plug-and-play)

Track A (Sensitive)

Mon: Session A

Wed: Session B

Fri: Session A (lighter volume)

Daily: 5–8 min mobility + walking baseline (split into short bouts if needed)

Track B (Steady)

Mon: Session A

Tue: mobility + walk

Thu: Session B

Sat: Session A or B (lighter)

Optional: one short “support session” (10–15 min) midweek: wall press + bridge + pillow squeeze

Track C (Athletic)

Mon: Session A (heavier)

Wed: Session B (control/lateral)

Fri: Phase 3 entry (load emphasis)

Sat or Sun: lighter single-leg session or carries + mobility

Running (if applicable): 2–3 easy sessions/week on non-heavy leg days

---

Progression rules (keep it boring, keep it effective)

Progress only after **3–5 stable days** and a good 24-hour response.

Pick **one** progression:

- +1 set to one main lift, OR
- +2 reps per set (within range), OR
- slightly more range (lower box by one notch), OR
- slightly less support (fingertips → one finger), OR
- small load increase (smallest available)

If you do not know what to progress, don't. Repeat the week and let adaptation catch up.

If you flare during the 30 days (do this immediately)

Use the Chapter 18 playbook, but here's the quick version:

Remove the newest progression (often step-downs, lateral lunges, extra walking, hills).

Switch strength for 3–7 days to **isometrics + short range**:

bridge hold, pillow squeeze, wall press, split-stance holds, higher box squat

Reduce walking by **20–40%** and keep it flat until baseline returns.

When stable for two days, return using **half-step progressions**.

Real-world examples (so you can actually follow this)

Desk worker

Biggest lever: movement interrupts + Track A/B schedule

Keep walks short but frequent; prioritize hinge + split stance to reduce back borrowing.

Walker/hiker

Biggest lever: walking baseline and hill control

Keep strength steady; add hills only after Week 2 is stable.

Runner

Biggest lever: keep run volume easy while Phase 2/3 builds control

If hip flares, reduce running dose first; keep strength consistent.

Lifter

Biggest lever: use box squats and hinges first; earn depth

Introduce load in Week 4 only if Week 3 was stable.

Quick checklist / Action plan

Choose Track A/B/C based on irritability and baseline stability.

Follow the week-by-week focus: Phase 1 → Phase 2 → Phase 2 capacity → consolidate/Phase 3 entry.

Use the guardrails: 0–3/10, no limping, 24-hour check, one dial at a time.

If you flare, step down immediately, don't wait for it to "prove" itself.

Reassess at Day 30: walking confidence, stairs, single-leg steadiness, and symptom predictability.

Chapter 20: Long-Term Hip Resilience

What this chapter will change for you

- You'll know how to keep hip pain from returning by maintaining **capacity, variety, and recovery**, without living in rehab forever.
- You'll learn the "minimum effective" weekly habits that protect your hips, back, and knees.
- You'll have a long-term progression strategy for walking, lifting, and running that prevents the boom–bust cycle.
- You'll build a simple personal operating system:

  baseline → build → consolidate → reset.

Resilience isn't "never feeling anything"

A resilient hip isn't a hip that never gets sore. It's a hip that:

- tolerates normal life and training without flaring

recovers quickly when it's challenged

stays strong across multiple directions (forward, sideways, rotation)

doesn't require constant micromanagement

The aim is not perfection. The aim is **adaptation**.

If hip pain taught you anything, it's that urgency and guesswork are expensive. Calm, consistent progression is cheaper and more reliable.

The four pillars of long-term hip health

Most long-term success comes from keeping these pillars alive.

Pillar 1: Capacity (strength that stays)

Hip strength fades if you stop loading it. Not immediately, but steadily.

Your hip needs ongoing exposure to:

- a squat pattern (sit-to-stand, squat, box squat)
- a hinge pattern (RDL, hip hinge, deadlift variation)
- a single-leg pattern (split squat, step-up, step-down)
- lateral and carry work (wall press, lateral lunge, suitcase carry)
- adductor support (slides, squeezes, lateral work that includes inner thigh)

You don't need all of this every session. You need it across the week.

Pillar 2: Variety (movement options)

Many flare-ups happen when your hip is asked to do a direction it hasn't practiced: deep flexion, rotation, hills, lateral movement.

Variety doesn't mean random workouts. It means you maintain a few motion options:

- gentle rotation
- tolerable extension exposure
- lateral weight shift

deep range only if earned and stable

Pillar 3: Dosage (load management you can live with)

The hip doesn't mind work. It minds spikes.

The long-term rule is simple: **don't change everything at once.**
If you increase running, keep lifting stable. If you increase lifting load, keep hills and sprints stable. You can build fast, but you must build predictably.

Pillar 4: Recovery (your tolerance ceiling)

Your tissues adapt when they recover. Poor sleep, high stress, illness, and travel reduce tolerance. The same workout becomes "too much" even if the plan hasn't changed.

Resilience includes knowing when your recovery is down and adjusting dose without drama.

Your minimum effective weekly plan (the "maintenance backbone")

This is for after the 30-day plan, when you want results to stick.

Option A: 2-day strength backbone (busy schedule)

Do two full-body hip-focused sessions per week.

Day 1 (squat + hinge + lateral)

Squat pattern: 3–4 x 5–8

Hinge pattern: 3–4 x 6–10

Suitcase carry: 3–5 x 20–40 sec/side

Optional adductor: towel slides 2 x 8/side

Day 2 (single-leg + step + rotation tolerance)

Split squat: 3 x 6–8/side

Step-up or step-down: 2–3 x 6–8/side

Lateral lunge (short range) OR wall press hold: 2–3 sets

Gentle hip rotations: 2 x 6/side

Walking: baseline daily movement (even 10–20 minutes) counts.

Option B: 3-day strength backbone (most people)

Day 1: Squat + hinge (heavier)

Day 2: Single-leg control (moderate)

Day 3: Lateral + carries + power entry (light/medium)

This keeps all directions trained without any single day becoming a punishment.

The "baseline → build → consolidate → reset" operating system

This is the long-term loop that prevents relapse.

1) Baseline (your stable floor)

Your baseline is what you can do consistently without next-day worsening:

walking time

weekly runs (if applicable)

strength volume

Baseline is not forever. It's a home base.

2) Build (small progressions)

Progress one dial at a time: load OR range OR speed OR volume.

A good build phase looks boring:

same movements

small increases

stable recovery

3) Consolidate (adaptation week)

Every 3rd–5th week, hold or slightly reduce volume. This is where tissues adapt and where many flare-ups are prevented.

Consolidation is not losing progress. It's locking it in.

4) Reset (when life hits)

Travel week, poor sleep, stressful period, your system needs a reset:

- keep strength at a minimum effective dose
- maintain walking/mobility
- reduce intensity temporarily
  Then return to baseline.

This is how resilient people train: they adjust without quitting.

Long-term walking, lifting, and running rules

Walking (for life)

- Keep a daily walking habit.
- Use hills as a training variable, not a surprise.
- If you increase hiking/steps, reduce gym volume that week.

Lifting (for resilience)

- Maintain hinges and single-leg work even when you're strong.
- Don't chase deep ranges under fatigue if your hip is flexion-sensitive.
- Use box squats or controlled depth as a tool, not a restriction.

Running (if you return)

- Keep at least one weekly single-leg strength day.
- Respect terrain: camber and hills are multipliers.
- Add speed last, and only after easy volume is stable for weeks.

Your early warning signs (catch problems before they flare)

Most flare-ups give warnings. Learn yours.

Common early signs:

- walking stride shortens unconsciously
- you start turning the foot out more
- stairs feel “grippy” in the front hip
- lateral hip ache appears sooner in a walk
- you feel the need to brace your back more than usual
- sleep quality drops and you feel “more sensitive”

If you notice these, don’t panic. Do a small reset:

- reduce volume by 20–30% for 3–7 days
- return to isometrics and short-range stability
- keep walking baseline but flatten terrain
- focus on breath + stack + hinge

Small resets prevent big setbacks.

The “forever” mobility plan (5 minutes, not 45)

You don’t need daily deep stretching. You need small, repeatable inputs that keep options open.

Pick 2–3 of these, most days:

- 90/90 supported rotations: 2 x 6/side
- standing back-step taps: 2 x 6/side
- adductor rock-backs (easy): 2 x 6/side
- gentle hip hinge to wall: 2 x 8
- supported single-leg stance: 2 x 20 sec/side

If you do just this, you’ll maintain a lot of what you rebuilt.

Common mistakes (and what to do instead)

Mistake: Stopping strength work once pain is gone

Instead: reduce to maintenance, don't eliminate. Capacity is your insurance policy.

Mistake: Switching to random workouts for "variety"

Instead: keep a stable backbone and add small, intentional variety (hills, speed, depth) one dial at a time.

Mistake: Ignoring recovery and blaming the hip

Instead: recognize when tolerance is down. Adjust dose calmly and return.

Mistake: Waiting for a flare-up to change your plan

Instead: respond to early warning signs with a small reset.

Quick checklist / Action plan

Keep a 2–3 day/week strength backbone (squat, hinge, single-leg, lateral/carries).

- Maintain a daily movement baseline (walking, short mobility).
- Progress one dial at a time and consolidate every 3rd–5th week.
- Use early warning signs to trigger a 3–7 day reset (reduce volume, keep supportive work).
- Remember the philosophy: calm, consistency, intelligent progression replaces urgency and guesswork.

Hip resilience isn't a special program you do once. It's a way of training and living that keeps your hip strong, adaptable, and trustworthy for years.

A Final Note from Evan Calder

If you've made it to the end of this book, you've already done something important: you stayed with a process long enough for your body to respond. That matters more than any single exercise.

Hip pain has a way of shrinking your world, shorter walks, avoided stairs, cautious training, a quiet fear of "setting it off." The work you've done here is the opposite of shrinking. You've rebuilt options. You've practiced calm exposure. You've increased capacity with a plan you can repeat.

Keep the philosophy close: **healing happens when calm, consistency, and intelligent progression replace urgency and guesswork.** When symptoms fluctuate, and they will at times, return to the fundamentals:

Set your **baseline**.

Train within **tolerance**.

Use the **24-hour check**.

Progress one dial at a time.

When needed, **step down early** and rebuild calmly.

There's no prize for forcing it. The win is a hip that feels more trustworthy month by month.

How to Use This Book Going Forward

If you're doing well and want to maintain

Use the **2–3 day/week strength backbone** from Chapter 20 and keep walking as your daily input. Rotate the patterns:

- squat pattern
- hinge pattern
- single-leg pattern
- lateral/carry pattern
- adductor support (light but consistent)

Reassess every 4–6 weeks with the mobility screen from Chapter 6. You're not chasing symmetry, you're checking that your options are still available.

If you're plateaued

Plateaus usually mean one of three things:

- Your baseline is still too high (you're living above tolerance).
- You're not progressing at all (you're underloading).
- You're progressing too many dials at once (you're spiking load).

Fix it by simplifying: choose one priority for 2–3 weeks (walk tolerance, single-leg control, or hinge strength) and progress one dial at a time.

If you flare

Re-read Chapter 18 and follow the playbook: **Settle → Protect → Maintain → Rebuild**.

Most flare-ups shrink quickly when you respond early and conservatively.

If a flare includes red flags (inability to bear weight, major trauma, fever, escalating night pain, new neurological symptoms), seek care.

Quick Reference: Your Decision Rules (One Page)

Pain and tolerance

Train in **0–3/10** discomfort and non-sharp sensations.

If pain climbs rep to rep, **scale the set**.

If you limp, **reduce dose**.

The 24-hour check

Better or the same tomorrow: continue (or progress if stable).

Worse tomorrow: reduce range first, then volume, then load.

Progression

Progress only after **3–5 stable days**, and change **one dial**:

range OR volume OR load OR speed

Regression (step-down)

When symptoms spike:

- remove the newest progression
- return to isometrics + short ranges for 3–7 days
- reduce walking volume 20–40% and keep flat

Exercise Index (by Goal)

Calm and reset

- breathing stack reset (Ch.5, 7, 18)
- gentle weight shifts (Ch.5, 18)

Mobility options

- supported hip rock-backs (Ch.5, 6, 8)
- 90/90 supported rotations (Ch.5, 6, 20)
- standing back-step taps (Ch.6, 8, 10)

Glute and lateral hip strength

bridge holds/reps (Ch.5, 7, 11)

side-lying abduction holds (Ch.7, 11)

lateral wall press holds (Ch.7, 11, 12)

suitcase carries (Ch.13, 20)

Adductors and pelvic stability

pillow squeeze isometrics (Ch.9, 11, 18)

towel slides (Ch.9, 12)

split-stance adductor bias hold (Ch.9)

Foundational patterns

sit-to-stand / box squat (Ch.5, 11, 14)

hip hinge to wall / RDL (Ch.11, 13, 16)

split-stance holds / split squats (Ch.11–14)

Single-leg control

supported single-leg stance (Ch.6, 12)

step-ups with slow lower (Ch.12, 17)

lateral step-downs (Ch.12, 17)

Running return tools

“shorter, quicker steps” cue (Ch.15)

flat baseline run/walk progressions (Ch.15)

Thank You for Reading

If this book helped you feel more confident in your body, calmer about movement, or clearer about what to do next, I'd be grateful if you shared your experience in a **short Amazon review**.

Your feedback helps other readers who may be living with pain, recovery, or uncertainty discover practical guidance they can trust. It also helps ensure these books continue to focus on what truly works in real life, clarity, patience, and steady progress.

Even a few honest words can make a meaningful difference.

Thank you for putting in the time, care, and consistency it takes to rebuild.

THE RECOVERY SERIES

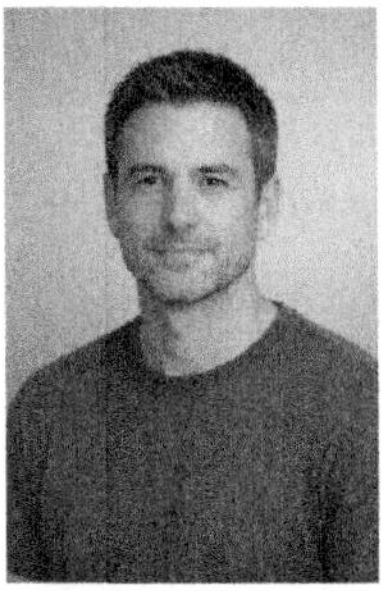

Evan Calder is a movement and recovery educator specializing in injury rehabilitation, physical resilience, and long-term strength for everyday people. His work focuses on helping readers rebuild confidence in their bodies after pain, injury, illness, or major life changes, without relying on extremes, shortcuts, or fear-based advice.

Website: **edenrootpress.com**
Instagram: **edenroot.press**

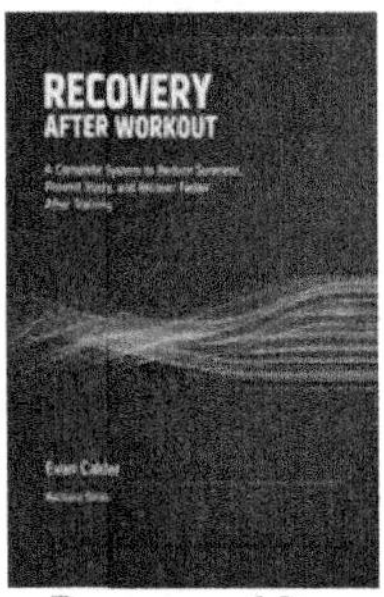

Recovery After Workout

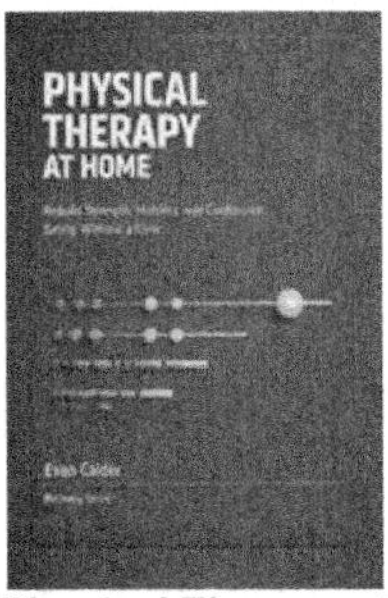

Physical Therapy at Home

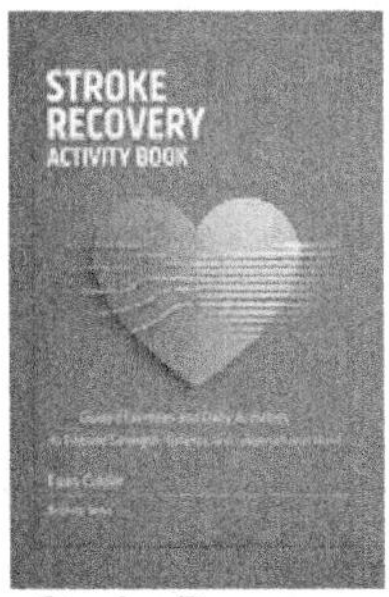

Stroke Recovery Activity Book

THE RECOVERY SERIES

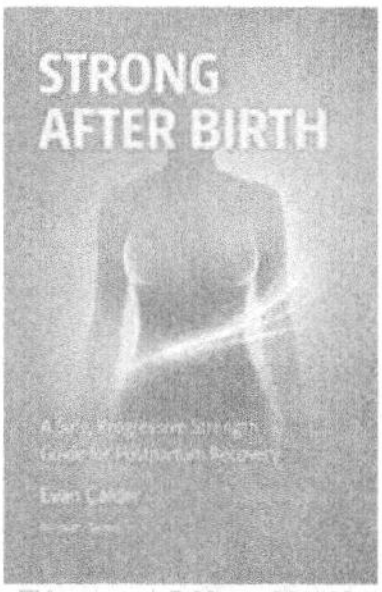

Strong After Birth

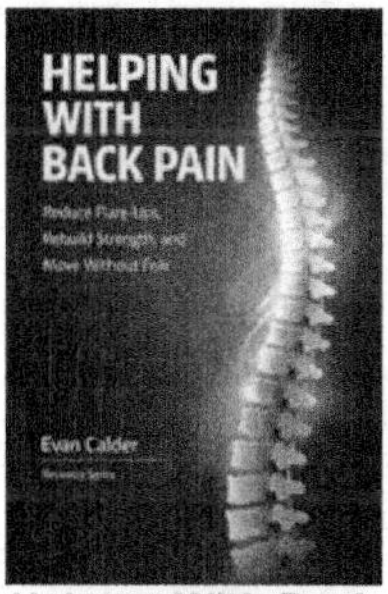

Helping With Back Pain

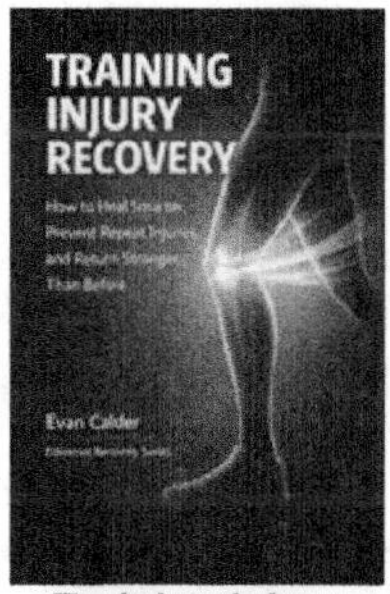

Training Injury Recovery

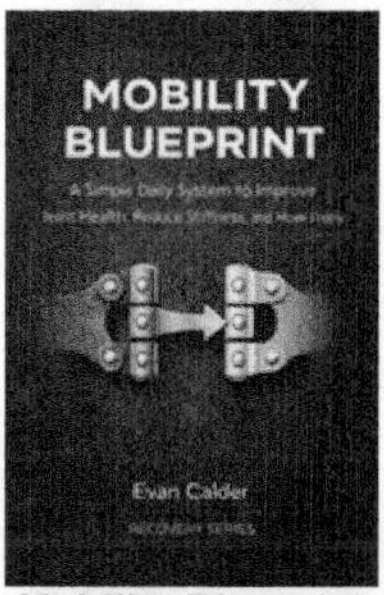

Mobility Blueprint

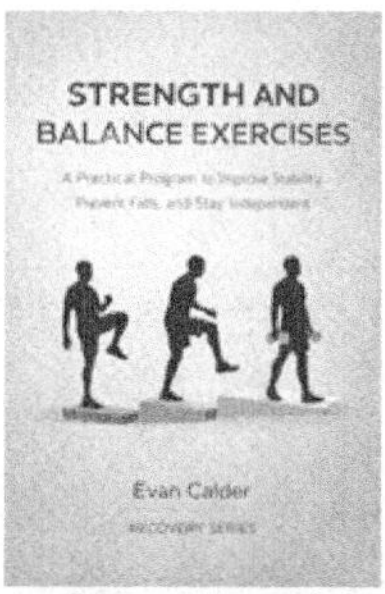

Strength and Balance Exercises

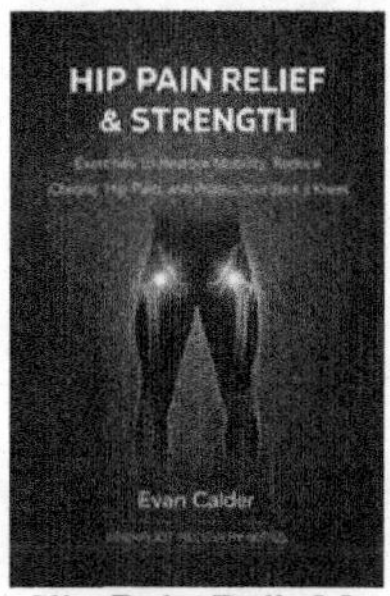

Hip Pain Relief & Strength

THE RECOVERY SERIES

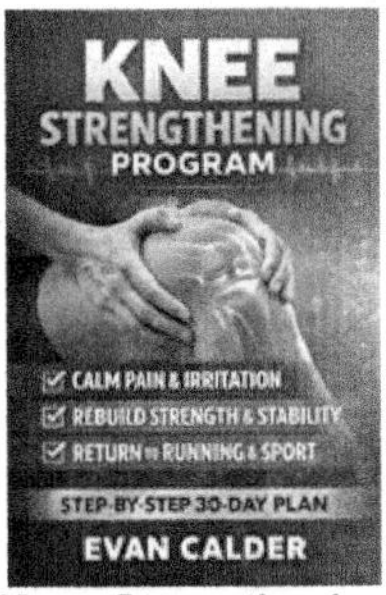

Knee Strengthening Program

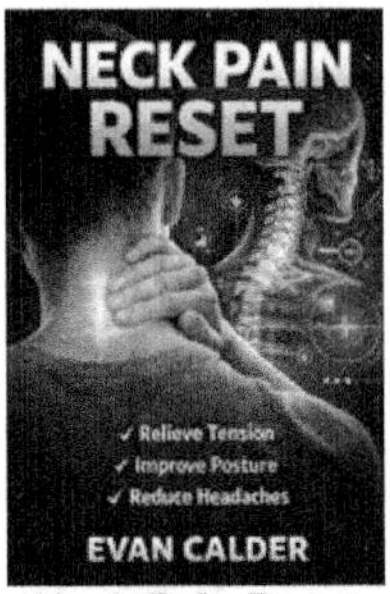

Neck Pain Reset

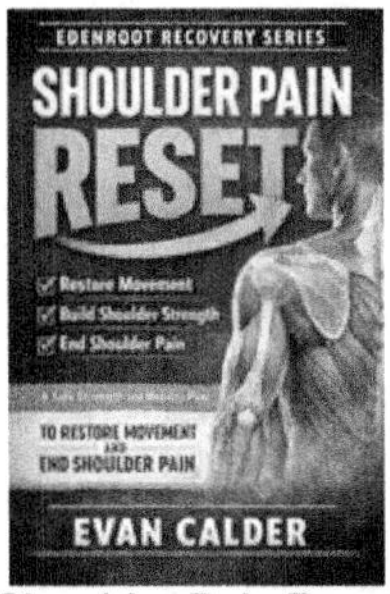

Shoulder Pain Reset

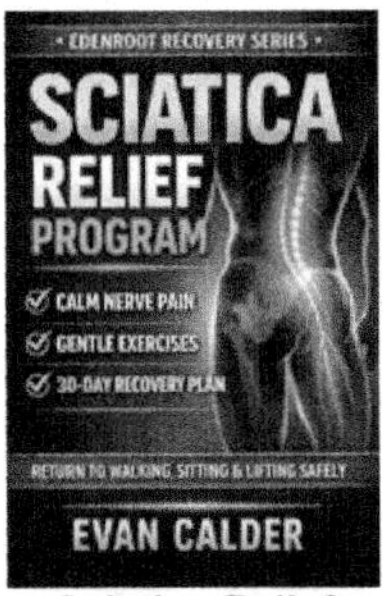

Sciatica Relief Program

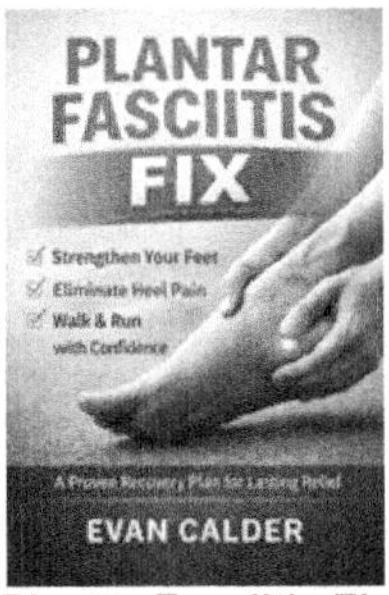

Plantar Fasciitis Fix

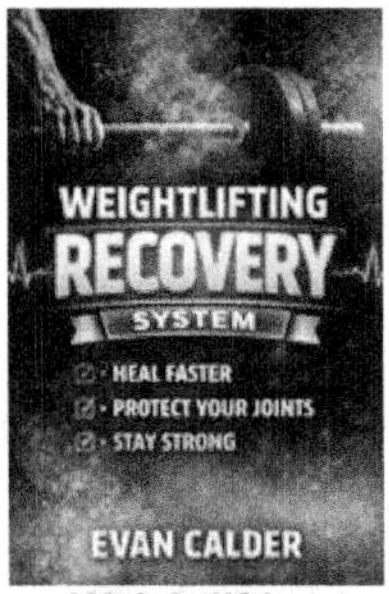

Weightlifting Recovery System

Printed in Dunstable, United Kingdom

78968276R00171